Hepatic Encephalopathy

Editor

VINOD K. RUSTGI

CLINICS IN LIVER DISEASE

www.liver.theclinics.com

Consulting Editor
NORMAN GITLIN

May 2020 • Volume 24 • Number 2

ELSEVIER

1600 John F. Kennedy Boulevard • Suite 1800 • Philadelphia, Pennsylvania, 19103-2899

http://www.theclinics.com

CLINICS IN LIVER DISEASE Volume 24, Number 2
May 2020 ISSN 1089-3261, ISBN-13: 978-0-323-68366-1

Editor: Kerry Holland
Developmental Editor: Donald Mumford

Clinics in Liver Disease (ISSN 1089-3261) is published quarterly by Elsevier Inc., 360 Park Avenue South, New York, NY 10010-1710. Months of issue are February, May, August, and November. Business and Editorial Offices: 1600 John F. Kennedy Blvd., Ste. 1800, Philadelphia, PA 19103-2899. Customer Service Office: 3251 Riverport Lane, Maryland Heights, MO 63043. Periodicals postage paid at New York, NY and additional mailing offices. Subscription prices are $313.00 per year (U.S. individuals), $100.00 per year (U.S. student/resident), $572.00 per year (U.S. institutions), $409.00 per year (international individuals), $200.00 per year (international student/resident), $709.00 per year (international instituitions), $343.00 per year (Canadian individuals), $100.00 per year (Canadian student/resident), and $709.00 per year (Canadian institutions). Foreign air speed delivery is included in all *Clinics* subscription prices. All prices are subject to change without notice. **POSTMASTER:** Send address changes to *Clinics in Liver Disease*, Elsevier Health Sciences Division, Subscription Customer Service, 3251 Riverport Lane, Maryland Heights, MO 63043. **Customer Service: Telephone: 1-800-654-2452 (U.S. and Canada); 314-447-8871 (outside U.S. and Canada). Fax: 314-447-8029. E-mail: journalscustomer service-usa@elsevier.com (for print support); journalsonlinesupport-usa@elsevier.com (for online support).**

Reprints. For copies of 100 or more of articles in this publication, please contact the Commercial Reprints Department, Elsevier Inc., 360 Park Avenue South, New York, NY 10010-1710. Tel.: 212-633-3874; Fax: 212-633-3820; E-mail: reprints@elsevier.com.

Clinics in Liver Disease is covered in *MEDLINE/PubMed (Index Medicus)*, Science Citation Index Expanded, Journal Citation Reports/Science Edition, and Current Contents/Clinical Medicine.

Contributors

CONSULTING EDITOR

NORMAN GITLIN, MD, FRCP (LONDON), FRCPE (EDINBURGH), FAASLD, FACP, FACG
Head of Hepatology, Southern California Liver Centers, San Clemente, California

EDITOR

VINOD K. RUSTGI, MD, MBA
Professor of Medicine, Clinical Director of Hepatology, Director, Center for Liver Diseases and Liver Masses, Professor of Epidemiology, Professor of Pathology and Laboratory Medicine, Rutgers Robert Wood Johnson Medical School, New Brunswick, New Jersey

AUTHORS

MARYAM ALIMIRAH, MD
Department of Internal Medicine, Henry Ford Hospital, Detroit, Michigan

MAGGIE CHEUNG, MD
Department of Internal Medicine, Rutgers Robert Wood Johnson Medical School, Department of Medicine, New Brunswick, New Jersey

PETER DELLATORE, MD
Department of Internal Medicine, Rutgers Robert Wood Johnson Medical School, Department of Medicine, New Brunswick, New Jersey

MOHAMED I. ELSAID, PhD, MPH, ALM
Research Education Specialist, Department of Medicine, Division of Gastroenterology and Hepatology, Rutgers Robert Wood Johnson Medical School, New Brunswick, New Jersey

PAUL J. GAGLIO, MD
Department of Medicine, Center for Liver Disease and Transplantation, NewYork-Presbyterian Hospital, Columbia University Medical Center, Columbia University Vagelos College of Physicians and Surgeons, New York, New York

FREDRIC D. GORDON, MD, FAASLD, FAST, AGAF
Vice Chair, Division of Transplantation and Hepatobiliary Diseases, Lahey Hospital and Medical Center, Burlington, Massachusetts; Associate Professor of Medicine, Tufts Medical School, Boston, Massachusetts

STUART C. GORDON, MD
Department of Gastroenterology and Hepatology, Henry Ford Hospital, Professor of Medicine, Wayne State University School of Medicine, Detroit, Michigan

ARIEL JAFFE, MD
Gastroenterology Fellow, Section of Digestive Diseases, Yale Liver Center, Yale School of Medicine, New Haven, Connecticut

SOFIA SIMONA JAKAB, MD
Associate Professor of Medicine, Section of Digestive Diseases, Yale Liver Center, Yale School of Medicine, New Haven, Connecticut; VA Connecticut Healthcare System, West Haven, Connecticut

TINA JOHN, MD, MPH
Department of Medicine, Division of Gastroenterology and Hepatology, Rutgers Robert Wood Johnson Medical School, New Brunswick, New Jersey

BRIETTE VERKEN KARANFILIAN, MD
Resident, Department of Internal Medicine, Rutgers Robert Wood Johnson Medical School, Department of Medicine, New Brunswick, New Jersey

ANITA KRISHNARAO, MD, MPH
Transplant Hepatology Fellow, Division of Transplantation and Hepatobiliary Diseases, Lahey Hospital and Medical Center, Burlington, Massachusetts

YOU LI, MS
Department of Medicine, Division of Gastroenterology and Hepatology, Rutgers Robert Wood Johnson Medical School, New Brunswick, New Jersey

JOSEPH K. LIM, MD
Professor of Medicine, Section of Digestive Diseases, Yale Liver Center, Yale School of Medicine, New Haven, Connecticut; VA Connecticut Healthcare System, West Haven, Connecticut

NOAH Y. MAHPOUR, MD
Medical Resident, Department of Internal Medicine, Rutgers Robert Wood Johnson Medical School, Department of Medicine, New Brunswick, New Jersey

TAEYANG PARK, MD
Resident, Department of Internal Medicine, Rutgers Robert Wood Johnson Medical School, Department of Medicine, New Brunswick, New Jersey

SRI RAM PENTAKOTA, MD, MPH, PhD
Department of Surgery, Rutgers New Jersey Medical School, Newark, New Jersey

LAUREN PIOPPO PHELAN, MD
Resident, Department of Medicine, Robert Wood Johnson University Hospital, Medical Resident, Department of Internal Medicine, Rutgers Robert Wood Johnson Medical School, New Brunswick, New Jersey

K. RAJENDER REDDY, MD
Ruimy Family President's Distinguished Professor of Medicine, Director of Hepatology, Division of Gastroenterology and Hepatology, Department of Medicine, University of Pennsylvania, Philadelphia, Pennsylvania

MISHAL REJA, MD
Medical Resident, Department of Internal Medicine, Resident, Department of Medicine, Robert Wood Johnson University Hospital, New Brunswick, New Jersey

RUSSELL ROSENBLATT, MD
Department of Medicine, Center for Liver Disease and Transplantation, NewYork-Presbyterian Hospital, Columbia University Medical Center, Columbia University Vagelos College of Physicians and Surgeons, New York, New York

VINOD K. RUSTGI, MD, MBA
Professor of Medicine, Clinical Director of Hepatology, Director, Center for Liver Diseases and Liver Masses, Professor of Epidemiology, Professor of Pathology and Laboratory Medicine, Rutgers Robert Wood Johnson Medical School, New Brunswick, New Jersey

OMAR SADIQ, MD
Department of Gastroenterology and Hepatology, Henry Ford Hospital, Detroit, Michigan

FRANK SENATORE, MD
Gastroenterology Fellow, Department of Gastroenterology and Hepatology, Rutgers Robert Wood Johnson Medical School, New Brunswick, New Jersey

AUGUSTINE TAWADROS, MD
Medical Resident, Department of Internal Medicine, Rutgers Robert Wood Johnson Medical School, Department of Medicine, New Brunswick, New Jersey

VANESSA WEIR, BA
Perelman Center for Advanced Medicine, Division of Gastroenterology and Hepatology, Department of Medicine, University of Pennsylvania, Philadelphia, Pennsylvania

JOHNATHAN YEH, PA
Department of Medicine, Center for Liver Disease and Transplantation, NewYork-Presbyterian Hospital, Columbia University Medical Center, Columbia University Vagelos College of Physicians and Surgeons, New York, New York

Contents

history and physical. Imaging is nonspecific; however, PET and MRI have shown areas of utility, but are not widely available, cost-efficient, or necessary for diagnosis. Electroencephalogram has shown promise as it can be used in conjunction with the Portal Systemic Hepatic Encephalopathy Score test to diagnose minimal HE. Further research on these techniques would need to be performed to identify strict criteria and cutoffs for diagnosing HE as well as associated sensitivities and specificities.

Briette Verken Karanfilian, Taeyang Park, Frank Senatore, and Vinod K. Rustgi

Minimal hepatic encephalopathy, previously called subclinical hepatic encephalopathy, represents the earliest and mildest form of hepatic encephalopathy. It is the most under-recognized and underdiagnosed form of hepatic encephalopathy. Although there is no diagnostic gold standard, validated testing modalities have been devised to detect this neurocognitive complication. The newest developments include medically related apps for smartphones or tablets that can be easily used to diagnose and monitor minimal hepatic encephalopathy. Although recognition of this neurocognitive impairment can be challenging, early detection is paramount with the discovery of an association with worse clinical outcomes in patients diagnosed with minimal hepatic encephalopathy.

Anita Krishnarao and Fredric D. Gordon

The presence of hepatic encephalopathy is often associated with worse clinical outcomes and increased mortality. Even subclinical hepatic encephalopathy has clinical impacts on daily life and has been linked to increased falls, motor vehicle accidents, and hospitalizations. The presence and degree of hepatic encephalopathy can also affect survival outcomes in cirrhosis, acute liver failure, and liver transplant recipients. Patients may have improved clinical outcomes after treatment of hepatic encephalopathy, but the long-term impact of treatment on prognosis is unclear.

Noah Y. Mahpour, Lauren Pioppo-Phelan, Mishal Reja, Augustine Tawadros, and Vinod K. Rustgi

Pharmacologic management of hepatic encephalopathy includes a broad range of therapies. This article covers the specific mainstays of therapies, such as antimicrobials and laxatives, with an established evidence base. This article also covers newer modalities of therapies, such as fecal microbiota transplant, probiotics, bioartificial support systems, small molecular therapies such as L-ornithine L-aspartate, branched chain amino acids, L-carnitine, zinc, and other forms of therapy currently under review.

Vanessa Weir and K. Rajender Reddy

Research increasingly shows that the gut-liver-brain axis is a crucial component in the pathophysiology of hepatic encephalopathy (HE). Due to the limitations of current standard-of-care medications, non-pharmacological treatments that target gut dysbiosis, including probiotics, nutritional management, and fecal microbiota transplants, are being considered as alternative and adjunct therapies. Meta-analyses note that probiotics could offer benefits in HE treatment, but have not shown superiority over lactulose. Emerging literature suggests that fecal microbiota transplants could offer a novel strategy to treat gut dysbiosis and favorably impact HE. Finally, liver support devices and liver transplantation could offer a last-resort treatment option for persistent HE.

Mohamed I. Elsaid, Tina John, You Li, Sri Ram Pentakota, and Vinod K. Rustgi

Hepatic encephalopathy is a major neuropsychiatric complication of liver disease that affects 30% to 40% of cirrhotic patients. Hepatic encephalopathy is characterized by a brain dysfunction that is associated with neurologic complications. Those complications are associated with cognitive impairments, which negatively impacts patients' physical and mental health. In turn, hepatic encephalopathy poses a substantial economic and use burdens to the health care system. This article reviews the multidimensional aspects of the health care burden posed by hepatic encephalopathy.

Russell Rosenblatt, Johnathan Yeh, and Paul J. Gaglio

Hepatic encephalopathy (HE) is a frequent indication for hospitalization and represents a common manifestation of portal hypertension and decompensated liver disease that contributes to hospital readmissions. Multiple new techniques are being evaluated to assist in preventing readmissions in these high-risk patients. Techniques to improve medication adherence are paramount. The use of telemedicine and on-demand patient assessment is likely to diminish hospitalizations for HE. Wearable technology has the potential to assist in HE diagnosis and prevent HE progression, with an anticipated diminution in hospital readmissions. This article discusses current and potential future techniques to improve outcomes in these vulnerable patients.

Mishal Reja, Lauren Pioppo Phelan, Frank Senatore, and Vinod K. Rustgi

Hepatic encephalopathy (HE) is a multifaceted disorder, with effects stretching far beyond office visits and hospitalizations. Patients with HE suffer from varying degrees of altered consciousness, intellectual disability, and personality changes. A large social impact exists for patients with HE. Quality of life and activities of daily living, such as work capacity, driving ability, and sleep quality, have been shown to be affected. Additionally, caregiver and financial burdens are highly prevalent. Multiple tools exist to assess quality of life, including the CLD-Q questionnaire. Common treatments for HE, including rifaximin and lactulose, have been shown to improve overall quality of life.

> Despite widespread use of lactulose and rifaximin for the treatment of hepatic encephalopathy, this complication of advanced liver disease remains a major burden on the health care system in the United States and continues to predispose to high morbidity and mortality. Several agents have surfaced over recent years with promise to treat hepatic encephalopathy and mitigate the cognitive impairment associated with this disease process. The purpose of this article is to highlight the leading emerging therapies in hepatic encephalopathy as well as their therapeutic targets.

CLINICS IN LIVER DISEASE

THE CLINICS ARE AVAILABLE ONLINE!
Access your subscription at:
www.theclinics.com

Preface

History of Hepatic Encephalopathy

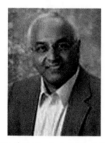

Vinod K Rustgi, MD, MBA
Editor

Hippocrates (460-371 BC) first recognized the relationship between the neuropsychological and physiologic changes observed in liver disease (**Figs. 1 and 2**). At that time, Hippocrates noted that there was a poor clinical outcome associated with delirium that was preceded by jaundice.[1]

Between 221 BC and 200 AD, the Qin-Han dynasties in Chinese medicine described the liver as having dynamic function connecting other organ systems via meridians.[2] According to ancient Chinese medicine, the liver housed an individual's spiritual consciousness that was responsible for emotion, communication, and expression.[3] The clinical manifestation of liver disease was a result of an imbalance within one or more of the meridians, which resulted in mental disorders, skin changes, and bleeding.[4]

In 700 AD, the Aztec people described illness as an imbalance between the souls: the tonalli, the teyolia, and the ihiyotl.[5] The ihiyotl soul resided in the liver, known to the Aztecs as *eltapachtli*. The ihiyotl was able to leave the body if it was summoned by a spiritual calling via the wind or an individual's breath.[6] The Aztecs observed that when individuals had an imbalance of the ihiyotl, they would become confused and agitated.[7] After the Spanish conquest of the Aztec Empire, there was a spread of endemic diseases between the 1600s and the late 1700s.[6] During this time, individuals would develop a yellow hue to their skin, fever, and confusion, and ultimately, die.[8] Autopsies conducted on these individuals found that their livers were pale and firm.[8]

As the clinical manifestations of hepatic encephalopathy became more prevalent throughout the world, there was an emergence of herbal remedies throughout China, India, and what is now Mexico. Traditional Chinese medicine evaluated each individual's manifestation of hepatic encephalopathy and determined an appropriate herbal treatment based on the afflicted organs, accumulation of toxins, and imbalanced yin-yang system.[3,4] Traditional Indian medicine (Ayurveda) was first practiced

Clin Liver Dis 24 (2020) xiii–xvii
https://doi.org/10.1016/j.cld.2020.02.001
1089-3261/20/© 2020 Published by Elsevier Inc.

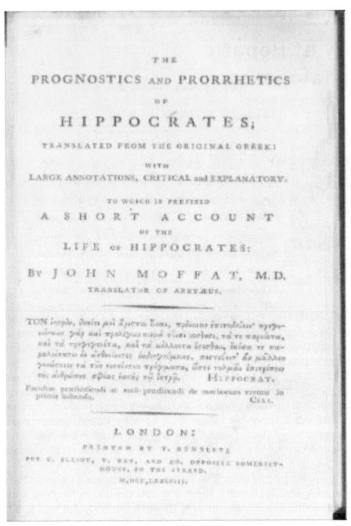

Fig. 1. "The Prognostics and Prorrhetics of Hippocrates" published in 1788.

3000 years ago and normalized liver function through a multifaceted approach of ingesting herbal remedies, nutrition, physical activity, and purification treatments.[9,10] The Aztec physicians, known as ticitl, used lippia dulcis, hojas de callito, and linaria to treat illnesses that were related to the liver.[6]

Although the clinical presentation of hepatic encephalopathy was described during the seventeenth and eighteenth centuries, the pathophysiology remained unclear until the early to mid-1900s.[11] During the 1940s and the 1950s, a number of advances were made in understanding the pathophysiology of hepatic encephalopathy. These developments came after a subgroup of individuals hospitalized in psychiatric facilities with delirium and mental status changes were found to have underlying liver disease.[12] This condition was termed portal-systemic encephalopathy and encompassed a clinical spectrum that was largely dependent on the cause of the liver disease.[11] It was noted that encephalopathy secondary to infectious hepatitis was rapid in onset with a worse

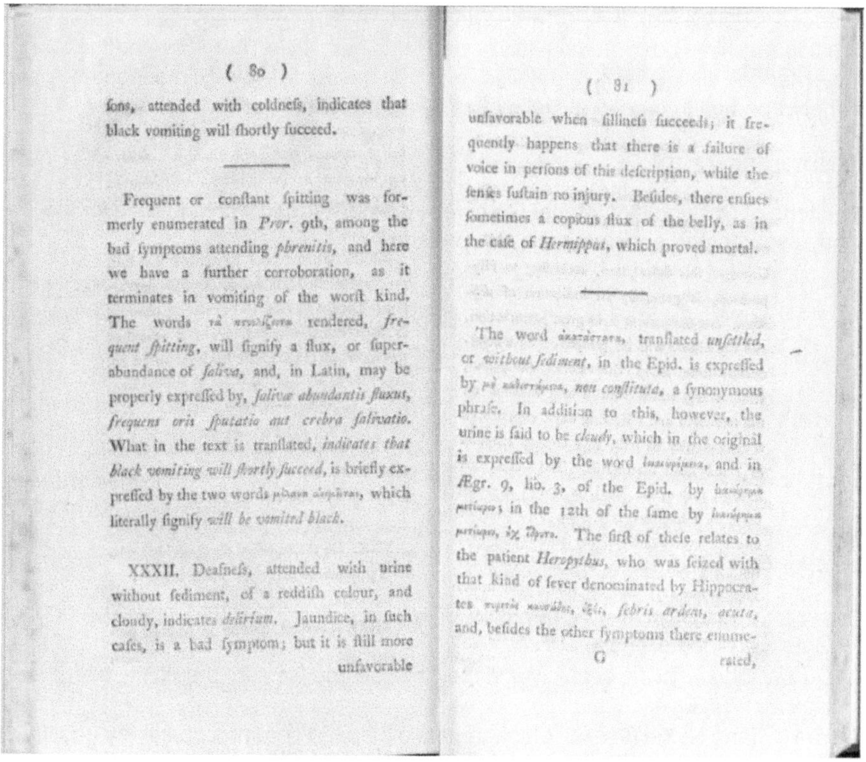

Fig. 2. Excerpt from "The Prognostics and Prorrhetics of Hippocrates" published in 1788 demonstrating the early understanding of hepatic encephalopathy.

prognosis, whereas encephalopathy secondary to portal cirrhosis was usually gradual in onset and sometimes precipitated by an inciting factor, such as gastrointestinal bleeding, infections, or toxin ingestion, and had the potential to be reversed.[13]

From the late 1950s to the mid-1960s, the role of ammonia was studied as a causative force driving the clinical syndrome of hepatic encephalopathy. It was hypothesized that the liver was unable to excrete ammonia from systemic circulation, and the accumulation of ammonia led to the clinical manifestation of hepatic encephalopathy.[14,15] The neurologic changes were thought in part to be due to excessive amounts of ammonia having direct access to the brain by way of large collateral portal vessels.[16]

However, many studies subsequently demonstrated that ammonia levels did not correlate with the degree of hepatic encephalopathy and that prompted further investigation into the role of ingested protein and bacterial activity in the gastrointestinal tract.[14,16-19] Managing gastrointestinal bleeding and reducing dietary intake of protein were routinely implemented to reduce the clinical burden of hepatic encephalopathy.[20] During the 1970s, it was found that the inability to manage toxic ammonia and ammine metabolites found in cirrhotic patients could be managed by antibiotics and enemas to decrease the bacteria and their production of ammonia from nitrogenous wastes within the gastrointestinal tract.[21,22]

Serial electroencephalographic (EEG) studies by the 1980s were able to detect delirium prior to clinical manifestations of hepatic encephalopathy.[23-25] EEGs were also used to correlate clinical improvement in hepatic encephalopathy due to the effects of antibiotics, enemas, and reduction of dietary protein.[23,26,27] In the last 3 decades, novel approaches to managing and evaluating patients with hepatic encephalopathy have been studied. It is hoped that this issue on hepatic encephalopathy will provide the clinician with a detailed review of the epidemiology, management, and its impact on health care in a succinct and enjoyable manner.

ACKNOWLEDGMENTS

The efforts of Dr Cynthia Vuittonet are hereby acknowledged with gratitude for the historical research and schematics in this preface.

Vinod K. Rustgi, MD, MBA
Center for Liver Diseases and Liver Masses
Rutgers Robert Wood Johnson Medical School
MedEd Building, Room 466
One Robert Wood Johnson Place
New Brunswick, NJ 08901, USA

E-mail address:
vr262@rwjms.rutgers.edu

REFERENCES

1. J. M. Prognostics and prorrhetics of Hippocrates translated from the original Greek. London: Bensley; 1788.
2. Liu ZW, Shu J, Tu JY, et al. Liver in the Chinese and western medicine. Integr Med Intnl 2017;4:39–45.
3. Yao C, Tang N, Xie G, et al. Management of hepatic encephalopathy by traditional Chinese medicine. Evid Based Complement Alternat Med 2012;2012:8.
4. Jia W, Gao WY, Yan YQ, et al. The rediscovery of ancient Chinese herbal formulas. Phytother Res 2004;18:681–6.
5. Olguin FRSs. The Aztec empire. New York: Guggenheim Museum Publications; 2004.
6. Torres E. Green medicine: traditional Mexican-American herbal remedies. Nieves Press; 1983.
7. Raymond GL. The Aztec god and other dramas. New York: G.P. Putnam's Sons; 1916.
8. Nicholson I. Mexican and central American mythology. New York: Bedrick Books; 1985.
9. Patel MV, Patel KB, Gupta S, et al. A complex multiherbal regimen based on Ayurveda medicine for the management of hepatic cirrhosis complicated by ascites: nonrandomized, uncontrolled, single group, open-label observational clinical study. Evid Based Complement Alternat Med 2015;2015:613182.
10. Kumar S, Dobos GJ, Rampp T. The significance of Ayurvedic medicinal plants. J Evid Based Complementary Alternat Med 2017;22:494–501.
11. Amodio P. Hepatic encephalopathy: historical remarks. J Clin Exp Hepatol 2015; 5:S4–6.
12. Sherlock S, Riddell AG, Summerskill WH, et al. Discussion on hepatic coma. Proc R Soc Med 1955;48:479–88.
13. Sherlock S. Emergencies in general practice: acute hepatic failure. Br Med J 1955;1:1383–5.
14. Najarian JS, Harper HA, McCorkle HJ. Recognition and treatment of alterations in ammonia metabolism. JAMA Surg 1959;79:621–9.

15. White LP, Phear EA, Summerskill WH, et al. Ammonium tolerance in liver disease: observations based on catheterization of the hepatic veins. J Clin Invest 1955;34: 158–68.
16. Summerskill WH, Davidson EA, Sherlock S, et al. The neuropsychiatric syndrome associated with hepatic cirrhosis and an extensive portal collateral circulation. Q J Med 1956;25:245–66.
17. Sherlock S. Pathogenesis and management of hepatic coma. Am J Med 1958;24: 805–13.
18. Sherlock S, Parbhoo SP. The management of acute hepatic failure. Postgrad Med J 1971;47:493–8.
19. Sherlock S. Hepatic encephalopathy. Br J Hosp Med 1977;17:144–6, 151-154, 159.
20. Sherlock S. Treatment of hepatic coma. Mod Treat 1969;6:131–41.
21. Riggio O, Ridola L, Pasquale C. Hepatic encephalopathy therapy: an overview. World J Gastrointest Pharmacol Ther 2010;1:54–63.
22. Antibiotics in hepatic coma. Br Med J 1958;1:512.
23. Bombardieri G, Gigli GL, Bernardi L, et al. Visual evoked potential recordings in hepatic encephalopathy and their variations during branched chain amino-acid treatment. Hepatogastroenterology 1985;32:3–7.
24. Hepatic encephalopathy: a unifying hypothesis. Nutr Rev 1980;38:371–3.
25. Electroencephalography in hepatic encephalopathy. JAMA 1963;184:209.
26. Larsen FS, Ranek L, Hansen BA, et al. Chronic portosystemic hepatic encephalopathy refractory to medical treatment successfully reversed by liver transplantation. Transpl Int 1995;8:246–7.
27. Loguercio C, Federico A, De Girolamo V, et al. Cyclic treatment of chronic hepatic encephalopathy with rifaximin. Results of a double-blind clinical study. Minerva Gastroenterol Dietol 2003;49:53–62.

Epidemiology of Hepatic Encephalopathy

Mohamed I. Elsaid, PhD, MPH, ALM[a],*, Vinod K. Rustgi, MD, MBA[b]

KEYWORDS

- Hepatic encephalopathy • Disease classification • Incidence • Prevalence
- Risk factors • Prevention

KEY POINTS

- In cirrhosis, the 1-, 5-, and 10-year cumulative incidence of HE ranges between 0% to 21%, 5% to 25%, and 7% to 42%, respectively.
- Within 2 years after transjugular intrahepatic portosystemic shunt (TIPS), the incidence of HE is between 20% and 55%.
- The prevalence ranges of minimal HE, HE in decompensated cirrhosis, and HE post-TIPS are 20% to 80%, 16% to 21%, and 10% to 50%, respectively.
- In cirrhosis, risk factors for overt HE include minimal HE, sarcopenia, hyponatremia, epilepsy, type 2 diabetes, high creatinine, high bilirubin, and low albumin.
- The development of either covert or overt HE is associated with poor survival of cirrhotic patients.

BACKGROUND

Hepatic encephalopathy (HE) is a common neuropsychiatric complication of both acute and chronic liver diseases.[1,2] Patients with HE usually experience a wide spectrum of cognitive impairments that range in severity from alterations of psychomotor speed and working memory to more progressive psychiatric manifestations, such as gross disorientation and coma.[3–7] As a result, HE is associated with significant economic and utilization burdens to patients and their caregivers.[8,9] The effects of HE extend beyond the direct economic and utilization impacts to include societal burdens related to patients' reduced quality of life and impairments in the activities of daily living.[5] The incidence of cirrhosis, the most common risk factor for HE, has steadily increased during recent years (**Fig. 1**).[10] Consequently, an upsurge in the clinical and health care burdens related to HE is expected in the upcoming years.

[a] Department of Medicine, Division of Gastroenterology and Hepatology, Rutgers Robert Wood Johnson Medical School, Medical Education Building, 1 Robert Wood Johnson, Room 479, New Brunswick, NJ 08903, USA; [b] Center for Liver Diseases and Liver Masses, Robert Wood Johnson School of Medicine, MedEd Building, Room 466, 1 Robert Wood Johnson Place, New Brunswick, NJ 08901, USA
* Corresponding author.
E-mail address: mie10@sph.rutgers.edu

Clin Liver Dis 24 (2020) 157–174
https://doi.org/10.1016/j.cld.2020.01.001
1089-3261/20/© 2020 Elsevier Inc. All rights reserved.

With that in mind, a comprehensive review of the epidemiology of HE has not been conducted to date. This review article aims to provide an overview of the epidemiology of HE.

DEFINITION

HE is characterized by the presence of hepatocellular failure, portosystemic shunting (PSS), or both.[7] In acute liver failure (ALF), abrupt loss of hepatocyte functions is associated with significant ammonia accumulations. Such accumulations result in hyperammonemia, which in turn can cause neuronal dysfunction, intracranial hypertension, cerebral edema, and HE.[2,11-13] The mechanisms underlining the onset of HE in cirrhosis are multifactorial. Primarily, the development of HE among cirrhotic patients was understood to be the direct effect of elevated levels of ammonia, which are shunted into the systemic circulation because of impaired liver function and hepatic decompensation. However, ammonia is currently identified as a risk factor for HE that is not sufficient for its diagnosis in cirrhosis.[14] Recent studies have identified other factors, such as inflammatory cytokines, manganese, benzodiazepine-like compounds, mercaptans, aromatic amino acids, and microbiota to be involved in the pathophysiology of HE.[2,15,16]

To reflect on its multidimensional pathophysiology, the American Association for the Study of Liver Disease (AASLD) and the European Association for the Study of the Liver (EASL) joint practice guideline defines HE as "A brain dysfunction caused by liver insufficiency and/or PSS; it manifests as a wide spectrum of neurological or psychiatric abnormalities ranging from subclinical alterations to coma."[7] According to this definition, HE is viewed as a broad range of negative alterations to behavioral, cognitive, or motor system functions that are caused by hepatic insufficiencies, perihepatic shunting, or both. In 2017, the International Society for Hepatic Encephalopathy and Nitrogen Metabolism (ISHEN) upheld the HE definition introduced by the AASLD/EASL practice guideline, and no further changes were proposed.[17]

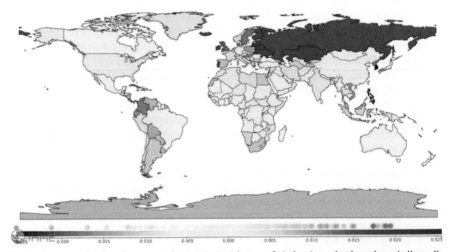

Fig. 1. Age-standardized percent change in incidence of cirrhosis and other chronic liver diseases, 1990 to 2017, new cases per 100,000. (*From* IHME. The Global Burden of Disease Study 2017 Institute for Health Metrics and Evaluation. Institute for Health Metrics and Evaluation Web site. http://vizhub.healthdata.org/gbd-compare/. Published 2018. Accessed 05/01, 2019. Institute for Health Metrics Evaluation. Used with permission. All rights reserved.)

CLASSIFICATION

The currently adopted approach to classifying HE is multiaxial as to reflect on the complex nature of the disease.[14,17] This multiparametric method was first put forward by the working party of the 11th World Congresses of Gastroenterology in their 1998 final report.[17,18] In 2011, the ISHEN implemented minor changes to the classification scheme introduced in 1998.[17] The updated scheme was then officially introduced in the joint AASLD/EASL practice guideline, and it is the currently followed method for HE classification. According to the AASLD/EASL guidelines, HE should be classified using 4 main axes: (1) the underlying cause, (2) the severity of the disease manifestation, (3) the time course of the disease, and (4) the existence of precipitating factors.[7] This 4-axial HE classification system ensures adequate patient management and standardized performance of observational studies and clinical trials.[17,18]

The Underlying Cause

The prognosis and management of HE differ based on the underlying disease pathophysiology.[19] In relation to disease cause, HE is classified into 3 subtypes. Type A is HE that develops as a result of ALF. HE caused by ALF is associated with osmotic disturbances in the brain, systemic inflammations, and elevated intracranial pressure that can cause cerebral herniation.[13] Hence, HE related to ALF signifies different prognosis and patient management requirements in comparison to HE related to chronic liver diseases. Although both type B and C share similar pathophysiology, the 2 subtypes have distinct prognoses.[14] Type B is HE associated with portal-systemic bypass or shunting in the absence of intrinsic liver dysfunction.[7,18] Type C, however, describes HE caused by cirrhosis, which is the most common risk factor for HE. Recent studies have shown that both the clinical and the pathophysiologic courses of HE differ in cirrhotic patients with versus without acute-on-chronic liver failure (ACLF).[20,21] In turn, it has been suggested that patients with HE related to ACLF should be classified as type D HE.[22]

The Severity of the Disease Manifestation

The severity of HE manifestations impacts both disease prognosis and treatment courses.[14] Classification of HE severity relies on 2 scales: the ISHEN grade and the West Haven criteria (WHC) (**Fig. 2**). The ISHEN grade makes a distinction between 2 types of HE: covert and overt.[7] Covert HE is characterized by signs of alterations to executive functions owing to brain dysfunction. Patients with covert HE show little to no clinical symptoms, and those affected do not require hospitalization.[19] In contrast, overt HE is marked by temporal and spatial disorientations or the presence of asterixis.[7,23] Clinical symptoms of overt HE are conspicuous, and they result in hospitalization.[19]

The WHC classification of HE includes 6 stages unimpaired, minimal and grades I through IV (see **Fig. 2**). Individuals with unimpaired HE do not experience any clinical or subclinical signs of HE.[7,23] Minimal hepatic encephalopathy (MHE) is the mildest form of disease onset, and it delineates subtle neurophysiologic alterations to cognitive functions detected by psychometric tests without any clinical evidence of mental changes.[7,18,24] Grade I HE is associated with cognitive and/or behavioral deteriorations in patients' regular performances on clinical examinations. From a clinical standpoint, differentiation between MHE and grade I HE is intangible. Finally, grades II through IV describe overt HE, and they range in severity from asterixis in grade II, to gross orientations in grade III, and coma in the case of grade IV.[7]

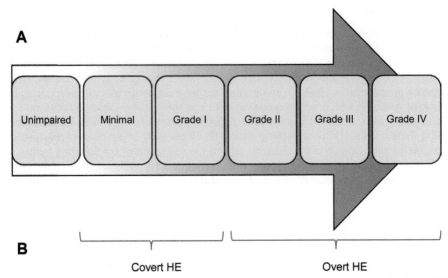

A

Unimpaired | Minimal | Grade I | Grade II | Grade III | Grade IV

B

Covert HE   Overt HE

Fig. 2. HE classification according to the severity of manifestation using (A) the WHC and (B) the ISHEN grade.[1] (*From* Vilstrup H, Amodio P, Bajaj J, et al. Hepatic Encephalopathy in Chronic Liver Disease: 2014 Practice Guideline by the European Association for the Study of the Liver and the American Association for the Study of Liver Diseases. *Journal of Hepatology.* 2014;61(3):642-659; with permission.)

According to Disease Time Course

Understanding the frequency of relapses in patients with HE aids in disease prognosis, in planning long-term management, and in guiding prophylactic treatments.[14,19,23] The time course of HE is divided into 3 intervals: episodic, recurrent, and persistent.[7] In the episodic interval, patients experience HE bouts more than 6 months apart.[23] Patients with recurrent HE suffer from bouts that take place within 6 months or less.[23] In the case of persistent HE, patients tend to experience unremitted behavioral modifications that are combined with relapses of overt HE bouts.[7]

The Existence of Precipitating Factors

The existence of precipitating factors is essential in diagnosing, confirming and determining the proper course of treatments for both episodic and recurrent HE (**Fig. 3**).[14,23] In relation to the presence of precipitating factors, HE is categorized into spontaneous (nonprecipitated) and precipitated.[7,23] Knowledge and treatment of precipitating factors could aid in recurrence preventions.[14] Namely, treating precipitating factors could resolve HE in 90% all patients.[7]

INCIDENCE

HE is a complex condition with multiple causes each with varied degrees of severity. The manifestations of HE range from clinically subtle signs, in the case of covert HE (ie, MHE or grade I HE), to coma, in the case of grade IV HE. At the same time, the use of multiple clinical tools in diagnosing HE impacts the comparability of measures of occurrences obtained from different studies.[7] Furthermore, multiple studies do not distinguish between the incidences of covert and overt HEs. As a result, quantifying precise incidence estimates for HE is a challenging task.[25,26]

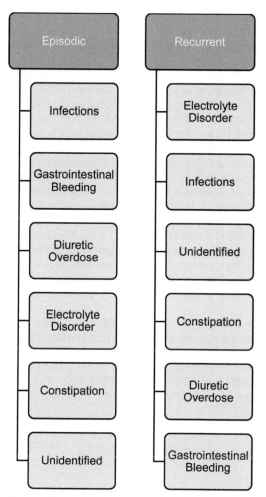

Fig. 3. Precipitating factors for episodic and recurrent overt HE by decreasing frequency. (*Adapted from* Vilstrup H, Amodio P, Bajaj J, et al. Hepatic Encephalopathy in Chronic Liver Disease: 2014 Practice Guideline by the European Association for the Study of the Liver and the American Association for the Study of Liver Diseases. *Journal of Hepatology.* 2014;61(3):642-659; with permission.)

The overall incidence of HE among cirrhotic patients has been reported in numerous studies. In the United States, an analysis of 186,481 Medicare patients with cirrhosis between 2008 and 2014 found the overall incidence of HE to be 26%, whereas the incidence rate of HE was 10.5 HE cases per 100 person-years.[27] Those estimates were comparable to results from a meta-analysis of 1200 cirrhotic patients in whom 22.0% of all subjects developed at least 1 HE bout with an average of 0.47 bouts per patient-year.[28] In the case of subclinical HE, the overall 48-month incidence of covert HE among cirrhotic patients in Mexico was 18.6%.[29] Those estimates were similar to a 17.5% overall MHE incidence reported by a study of 196 patients with cirrhosis in northern India.[30]

Several analyses showed that the incidence of HE depends on the type and severity of the primary hepatic insufficiencies.[7] The 5-year incidence of overt HE in cirrhotic patients ranges between 5% and 25% depending on the underlying cause and the presence of complications.[7,31] Similar variations in the 1- and 10-year incidence estimates have been reported in multiple studies. In a cohort analysis of 1317 Swedish patients with cirrhosis, both the 1- and 10-year cumulative incidences of HE differed by cause (**Fig. 4**).[32] Between 2001 and 2017, the overall incidence of HE was 33%. The 1-year cumulative incidence of HE was between 0% and 21%, whereas the maximum and minimum 10-year cumulative incidences were 7% and 42%, respectively. Patients with alcoholic cirrhosis had the highest risk of HE, whereas the 1- and 10-year cumulative HE incidences among patients with decompensated cirrhosis were 6.4% and 26%, respectively.

The association between viral hepatitis and the incidence of HE in cirrhosis was investigated in 2 Italian studies. In a cohort study of 312 Italian patients with compensated cirrhosis owing to hepatitis B or C, the overall incidence of HE was 1.9%, whereas the 5- and 10-year cumulative incidences were 0% and 5.0%, respectively.[33] During follow-up, the incidence of HE was slightly higher in patients with hepatitis B compared with those with hepatitis C (2.3% vs 1.9%). However, in a longitudinal study of the natural history of viral hepatitis–induced cirrhosis, Gentilini and colleagues[34] reported higher HE incidence estimates compared with those obtained by Benvegnu and colleagues.[33] Among hepatitis-induced cirrhotic patients, Gentilini and colleagues found the 5-, 10-, and 15-year cumulative HE incidences to be 9.1%, 25.6%, and 54.5%, respectively.

Based on patients' demographics and the disease definition used, the overall incidence of HE following transjugular intrahepatic portosystemic shunt (TIPS) is between 18% and 45%.[35] Studies have found the incidence of refractory HE post-TIPS to range between 3% and 8%.[35] In a retrospective study of 191 patients, the 30-day cumulative incidence of HE was 42% post-TIPS, with 46%, 29%, 18%, and 7% of patients with incident HE having grades I, II, III, and IV, respectively.[36] Within 2-years post-TIPS, studies

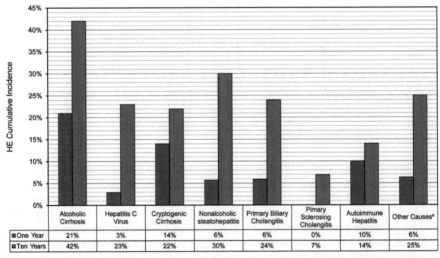

	Alcoholic Cirrhosis	Hepatitis C Virus	Cryptogenic Cirrhosis	Nonalcoholic steatohepatitis	Primary Biliary Cholangitis	Pimary Sclerosing Cholangitis	Autoimmune Hepatitis	Other Causes[a]
One Year	21%	3%	14%	6%	6%	0%	10%	6%
Ten Years	42%	23%	22%	30%	24%	7%	14%	25%

Fig. 4. Cumulative incidence of HE by cause of cirrhosis in 1317 cirrhotic patients, 2001 to 2017. [a] Other causes of cirrhosis included hepatitis B, hemochromatosis, and alfa-1 antitrypsin deficiency. (*Adapted from* Nilsson E, Anderson H, Sargenti K, Lindgren S, Prytz H. Clinical course and mortality by etiology of liver cirrhosis in Sweden: a population based, long-term follow-up study of 1317 patients. *Alimentary Pharmacology & Therapeutics.* 2019;49(11):1421-1430; with permission.)

reported the incidence of HE to range between 20% and 55%.[37–39] One-year post-TIPS, Schepis and colleagues[40] found the incidence of HE to be 27% and 54% among patients with underdilated polytetrafluoroethylene-covered stent-grafts (PTFE-SGs) TIPS (ie, 7 and 6 mm) and those who received PTFE-SGs TIPS of 8 mm or more, respectively. The incidence of post-TIPS HE in 70 patients with recurrent variceal hemorrhage was reported in 1 study to be 42.8%,[37] whereas the pooled post-TIPS cumulative incidence of HE among patients with hepatorenal syndrome was 49%.[41]

PREVALENCE

As it is the case with incidence estimates, data on the prevalence of HE vary depending on the underlying cause, severity of the disease manifestation, and the definition of HE (covert vs overt). Among patients with cirrhosis, the prevalence of subclinical HE (ie, MHE or covert HE) ranges between 20% and 80%.[30,31,42–48] The prevalence of covert HE, in a Chinese study of 336 cirrhotic patients, was 35.8%.[49] At the time of first cirrhosis diagnosis, the prevalence of overt HE is between 10% and 20%.[50–52] In decompensated cirrhosis, the prevalence of overt HE ranges between 16% and 21%.[7] In a study of cirrhotic patients pre-TIPS and post-TIPS, the prevalence of HE was 6.1% and 15.6% during the 6 months and 15 months postoperatively.[53] Other studies noted that the overall prevalence of HE in patients with TIPS is between 10% and 50%.[7] With all that in mind, an estimated 30% to 40% of cirrhotic patients will experience overt HE during the clinical course of their illnesses.[7,54]

RISK FACTORS OF OVERT HEPATIC ENCEPHALOPATHY
Posttransjugular Intrahepatic Portosystemic Shunt

TIPS plays an essential role in the treatment of portal hypertension complications, including variceal bleeding and refractory ascites. However, TIPS results in a significant increase in the risk of postprocedural overt HE.[55,56] Such an increase in the risk of HE occurrence post-TIPS is associated with several factors, including older age,[36,38,39,57–59] higher Child-Pugh score,[38,57] higher model of end-stage liver disease (MELD) score,[36,59–61] prior history of HE pre-TIPS,[38,57,59] low portosystemic pressure gradient (PPG),[57,61–63] proton pump inhibitor (PPI) use,[59,64] refractory ascites,[65] and underdilated TIPS.[40] Risk factors associated with refractory HE post-TIPS include prior history of HE pre-TIPS, the shunt size (>8 mm vs ≤ 8 mm), low serum albumin, and high creatinine levels.[35,39]

The effects of age were noted in a cohort study of 78 patients with cirrhosis treated by TIPS using PTFE-SGs. In this study, a 1-year increase in age was associated with adjusted hazard ratio (aHR) 1.09 (95% confidence interval [CI]: 1.05, 1.13) higher risk of HE occurrence post-TIPS.[39] Those findings were similar to results from 2 observational studies where a 1-year increase in age was associated with adjusted incidence rate ratio (aIRR) of 1.05 (95% CI%: 1.03, 1.07),[59] and aHR 1.05 (95% CI%: 1.02, 1.08)[38] increases in the risk of HE postoperatively.

Several studies have shown that both the Child-Pugh and the MELD scores are independently associated with increased risk of HE development post-TIPS. A unit increase in the Child-Pugh score has been shown in an observational study to increase the risk of HE post-TIPS by 29%.[38] Those findings were comparable to the pooled estimates obtained from a meta-analysis of 4 studies.[57] Three observational studies reported that a 1-unit increase in the MELD score is associated with 1.70 (95% CI: 1.39, 2.06) higher odds of HE post-TIPS, 1.16 (95% CI: 1.01, 1.34) -fold increase in the risk of HE following TIPS, and 1.06 (95% CI: 1.01, 1.11) times the HE aIRR after TIPS.[59–61]

History of HE before TIPS is a significant predictor of HE development postprocedurally. In a meta-analysis of 11 studies, patients with prior history of HE pre-TIPS had 3.07 (95% CI: 1.75, 5.40) higher odds of HE post-TIPS compared with those without prior history of HE pre-TIPS.[57] In a retrospective study of 284 patient, the aIRR of new or worsening HE post-TIPS was 1.51 (95% CI: 1.04, 2.20) higher for patients with versus those without history of HE or HE prophylactic pre-TIPS.[59] A prospective analysis of 82 consecutive cirrhosis patients reported a 3.16 (95% CI: 1.43, 6.99) increase in the risk of HE occurrence post-TIPS for patients with covert HE pre-TIPS versus those without HE pre-TIPS.[38]

Portal vein pressure reduction by TIPS is essential to improving the symptoms of portal hypertension; however, pressure that is too low could increase the risk of HE postoperatively.[7,66,67] A study of 210 patients treated with TIPS reported a significantly higher hepatic venous pressure gradient (HVPG) difference (ie, initial HVPG − final HVPG) for those with versus those without post-TIPS HE (10.5 mm Hg vs 8.9 mm Hg, $P = .030$).[62] In a study of 279 patients with hepatocellular carcinoma, a 1-mm Hg decrease in post-TIPS PPG was associated with 1.20 (95% CI: 1.07, 1.33) -fold increase in the risk of HE postprocedurally.[61] Similar findings of higher risk of HE post-TIPS in relation to higher PPG were reported in a systemic review of 30 papers.[57]

Several studies have been conducted to investigate the impact of PPI, refractory ascites, and underdilated TIPS on the risk of HE development postoperatively. In a recent study of 284 patients, PPI use was associated with increased risk of HE post-TIPS. In this study, patients with chronic use of PPI pre-TIPS had 3.19 (95% CI: 2.19, 4.66) times the hazard of HE post-TIPS compared with those without PPI use.[59] In a multivariate analysis using data on 54 patients with TIPS, the incidence of HE postprocedurally was almost doubled in patients with refractory ascites versus those without (89% vs 46%; $P<.001$).[65] Underdilated TIPS (ie, 7 and 6 mm) was shown in a prospective, nonrandomized study of cirrhotic patients to be associated with a lower risk of HE compared with patients who received PTFE-SGs of 8 mm or more (27% vs 54%, $P = .015$).[40]

In Cirrhosis

The presence of overt HE in cirrhotic patients signifies the decompensated stage of the disease.[7] A predominant proportion of both episodic and recurrent overt HE cases occurs in response to onsets of several precipitating factors (**Fig. 5**).[7,68,69] The most common precipitating factors in episodic HE are infections, which include spontaneous bacterial peritonitis, urinary tract infections, respiratory infections, skin infections, and sepsis.[19,29] In addition to the presence of precipitating factors, several studies have identified multiple risk factors that can lead to HE development or reoccurrence.[27,29,70–80] In cirrhosis, major risk factors for overt HE include MHE, prior history of overt HE, sarcopenia, hyponatremia, epilepsy, type 2 diabetes mellitus (T2DM), higher creatinine levels, higher bilirubin levels, lower levels of albumin, PPI use, nonselective beta-blockers use, and statin use.

The presence of MHE has been associated with disease severity and increases in both the annual and the cumulative rates of cirrhosis progressions.[70] In turn, MHE is considered to be one of the main risk factors for overt HE.[81] In a study of 68 patients with cirrhosis, those with MHE at baseline had an aHR 2.02 (95% CI: 1.23, 3.33) times the risk of overt HE compared with those without MHE.[78] In a prospective study of 116 histology-proven cirrhosis patients, the presence of subclinical HE was associated with a 3.70-fold increase in the risk of developing overt HE.[31] Those results were similar to findings from a later prospective study of 310 cirrhotic patients in whom

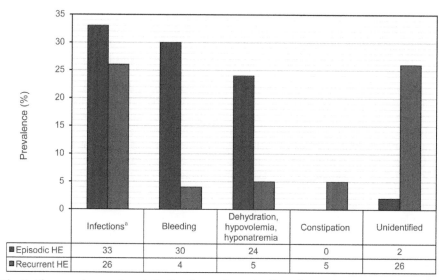

	Infections[a]	Bleeding	Dehydration, hypovolemia, hyponatremia	Constipation	Unidentified
■ Episodic HE	33	30	24	0	2
■ Recurrent HE	26	4	5	5	26

Fig. 5. The prevalence of precipitating factors for episodic and recurrent HE. [a] Spontaneous bacterial peritonitis, urinary infections, respiratory infections, sepsis (unknown), and skin infections. (*Adapted from* Amodio P. Hepatic encephalopathy: Diagnosis and management. *Liver International.* 2018;38(6):966-975; and Strauss E. The importance of bacterial infections as precipitating factors of chronic hepatic encephalopathy in cirrhosis. *Hepato-gastroenterology.* 1998;45(21):900-904.)

the risk of overt HE was 1.79 (95% CI: 1.21, 2.65) in those with versus those without MHE.[82]

Multiple studies have noted that prior history of HE is an independent risk factor for HE reoccurrence in cirrhosis.[75,76,78,82,83] In an open-label randomized controlled trial of 125 cirrhosis patients with resolved HE, 33.6% of all individuals experienced an overt HE episode during a median follow-up period of 14 months.[83] A prospective study of 310 patients with cirrhosis reported similar results of increased risk of HE for those with versus those without prior history of overt HE, aHR 2.45 (95% CI: 1.66, 3.58).[82] The number of prior HE episodes has also been shown to be directly associated with the risk of subsequent HE bouts, whereby each additional prior HE episode increases the risk of a consequent HE bout by 23%.[71]

Comorbid conditions that independently increase the risk of overt HE development include sarcopenia, hyponatremia, T2DM, and epilepsy. In a meta-analysis of 6 observational studies, the pooled odds of HE presence for sarcopenia patients were 2.74 (95% CI: 1.87, 4.01) times the odds for those without sarcopenia.[72] The role of hyponatremia as a risk factor for HE development was evaluated in several studies. In a prospective study, having hyponatremia (serum sodium <130 mEq/L) was associated with an aHR 10.69 (95% CI: 4.39, 26.03) higher risk of HE, whereas a retrospective analysis noted 1.35 (95% CI: 1.04, 1.75) times the risk of HE development for hyponatremia patients versus those without hyponatremia.[74,75]

A study of the relationship between T2DM and HE found the aHR for first-time overt HE occurrence to be 1.86 (95% CI: 1.20, 2.87) for diabetics compared with nondiabetics.[77] Moreover, in a secondary analysis, the risk of HE among those with diabetes was an aHR 1.41 (95% CI: 1.09, 1.82) times the risk for nondiabetics.[76] Those findings were consistent with results from a study of patients with hepatitis C virus–related cirrhosis in whom greater severity of HE was associated with the presence of dia-betes.[80] The effects of epilepsy on the risk of HE development were evaluated in a secondary analysis of data from 3 randomized trials.[76] The analysis found epilepsy to be associated with a significant increase in the risk of overt HE (grade II through IV) aHR 3.83 (95% CI: 1.65, 8.87).[76] However, the relationship was not statistically sig-nificant when HE was defined as grades I through IV, aHR of 2.12 (95% CI: 0.99, 4.55).

Changes in the levels of bilirubin, albumin, and creatinine have been independently associated with increases in the risk of HE development in cirrhotic patients (**Table 1**).[29,74–79,82] In a retrospective study of 1979 cirrhotic patients, an increase of 1 mg/dL in bilirubin level was associated with a 7% increase in the risk of HE.[79] Sim-ilarity, the presence of hyperbilirubinemia significantly increased the risk of HE in 2 cohort studies.[74,75] Findings from 2 cohort analyses of 2289 showed that a 1-mg/dL increase in albumin level reduces the risk of HE by 46% to 53%.[79,82] Four different observational studies that included a total of 1213 patients with cirrhosis noted that higher levels of creatinine increase the risk of HE.[29,74,75,77]

Three different studies investigated the relationship between PPI and HE in cirrhosis.[27,73,82] All 3 studies found a direct association between PPI use and increased risk of HE that ranged between 36% and 83%. In a retrospective cohort study of veter-ans in the United States, nonselective beta-blockers were associated with a 34% in-crease in the risk of HE, whereas statin use reduced the risk of HE by 20%.[27]

SURVIVAL IN HEPATIC ENCEPHALOPATHY

The development of HE is associated with poor survival in cirrhotic patients.[84,85] Such low survival is not only limited to the occurrence of overt HE, but patients with covert HE also experienced higher risks of mortality.[49,51,86,87] In a prospective study of 117 patients with cirrhosis, individuals with MHE (defined as critical flicker frequency <39 Hz) had significantly lower survival rates compared with those without MHE (MHE vs no MHE; 68.6% vs 82%; $P = .024$).[88] Compared with those free of MHE, hav-ing MHE remained a significant predictor of higher mortality in the multivariable anal-ysis with an aHR of 4.36 (95% CI: 1.67, 11.37). Patidar and colleagues[89] followed 170 cirrhotic patients for 13.0 ± 14.6 months to evaluate their survival and hospitalization rates. In this study, the 1-, 2-, 3-, and 4-year cumulative incidences for mortality or liver transplantation were 2.6% vs 17.6%, 10.1% vs 20.4%, 22.5% vs 54.3%, and 22.5% vs 75.6%, respectively, for subjects without covert HE versus patients with covert HE. One and 5 years following the first bout of acute HE, cirrhotic patients have survival probabilities of only 42% and 23%, respectively.[84] The 1- and 5-year survival rates of alcoholic cirrhosis-related patients with overt HE is 36% and 15%, respectively.[51]

TIPS improves the survival of cirrhotic patients awaiting liver transplantation.[90] At the same time, TIPS more than doubles the risk of HE postoperatively compared with stan-dard endoscopic interventions.[55,90] Patients with HE undergoing TIPS experience a higher mortality risk postprocedurally. In a study of 68 patients treated by TIPS, patients with pre-TIPS HE had more than a 3-fold increase in the risk of death 1 year postoper-atively.[91] Those findings were similar to results from a study of 223 patients with end-stage liver disease who underwent TIPS.[85] Risk factors for increased risk of mortality in HE include older age, high bilirubin levels, increase in creatinine levels, HE grade (III–IV vs I–II), PPI use, prior history of HE, MHE, and higher MELD score.[20,82]

PREVENTION OF OVERT HEPATIC ENCEPHALOPATHY

The primary strategy for managing overt HE includes secondary prophylaxis for recur-rence prevention.[92] In a meta-analysis of 24 randomized clinical trials, the use of

Table 1
Summary of main studies reporting the associations between the risk of hepatic encephalopathy and levels of bilirubin, albumin, and creatinine in cirrhotic patients

Exposure	Author (y)	Sample Size	Study Design	Measure of Association	Estimate (95% CI)
Bilirubin, comparison unit					
≥ 2.1 mg/dL vs <2.1 mg/dL	Guevara et al,[75] 2009	61	Prospective cohort	Adjusted hazard ratio	2.74 (1.16–6.47)
≥1.9 mg/dL vs <1.9 mg/dL	Guevara et al,[74] 2010	70	Retrospective cohort	Adjusted hazard ratio	1.87 (1.35–2.59)
Per 10 μmol/L increase	Jepsen et al,[77] 2015	862	Secondary analysis[a]	Adjusted hazard ratio	1.06 (1.03–1.08)
Per 1 mg/dL increase	Tapper et al,[79] 2018	1979	Retrospective cohort	Adjusted hazard ratio	1.07 (1.05–1.09)
Albumin					
Per 5 g/L increase	Jepsen et al,[77] 2015	862	Secondary analysis[a]	Adjusted hazard ratio	0.68 (0.56–0.83)
Per 5 g/L increase	Jepsen et al,[76] 2016	1120	Secondary analysis[a]	Adjusted hazard ratio	0.78 (0.70–0.87)
<3.5 g/dL vs ≥3.5 g/dL	Riggio et al,[78] 2015	216	Retrospective cohort	Adjusted hazard ratio	2.60 (1.36–4.97)
Per 1 mg/dL increase	Tapper et al,[79] 2018	1979	Retrospective cohort	Adjusted hazard ratio	0.54 (0.48–0.59)
Per 1 g/L increase	Nardelli et al,[82] 2019	310	Prospective cohort	Adjusted hazard ratio	0.47 (0.33–0.69)
Creatinine					
≥ 1.2 mg/dL vs <1.2 mg/dL	Guevara et al,[75] 2009	61	Prospective cohort	Adjusted hazard ratio	2.36 (1.11–5.00)
≥ 1.3 mg/dL vs <1.3 mg/dL	Guevara et al,[74] 2010	70	Retrospective cohort	Adjusted hazard ratio	1.48 (1.11–1.96)
Per 10 μmol/L increase	Jepsen et al,[77] 2015	862	Secondary analysis[a]	Adjusted hazard ratio	1.09 (1.05–1.13)
Per 1 mg/dL increase	Ruiz-Margáin et al,[29] 2016	220	Prospective cohort	Adjusted hazard ratio	4.11 (1.57–10.77)

[a] Included data from 3 clinical trails.
Data from Refs.[29,74–79,82]

nonabsorbable disaccharides (ie, lactulose or lactitol) was associated with a 42% reduction in the risk of HE occurrence or reoccurrence compared with placebo or no intervention.[93] Treatment with lactulose or lactitol, compared with placebo or no intervention, was also associated with a 41% drop in mortality risk and a 53% reduction in the rate of liver-related serious events. In a placebo-controlled trial, whereby 90% of both groups received concomitant lactulose, rifaximin use was associated with 58% reduction in the risk of HE reoccurrence after the first overt HE bout.[94] Other trials found similar results of high effectiveness of rifaximin plus lactulose in maintaining remission in cirrhotic patients with HE.[7] Thus, combination therapy of rifaximin and lactulose is the AASLD/EASL-recommended treatment for the prevention of overt HE reoccurrence among cirrhotic patients. In contrast, there is no evidence to support the use of rifaximin or lactulose as prophylactic agents for preventing HE reoccurrence post-TIPS.

SUMMARY

HE is a common neuropsychiatric complication of both acute and chronic liver diseases. The onset of HE is associated with a broad range of negative alterations to behavioral, cognitive, or motor system functions that are caused by hepatic insufficiencies, perihepatic shunting, or both. To ensure adequate patient management and standardized performance of observational studies and clinical trials, HE is classified using 4 main axes: (1) the underlying cause, (2) the severity of the disease manifestation, (3) the time course of the disease, and (4) the existence of precipitating factors. Quantifying precise incidence and prevalence measures for HE is challenging because of differences in cause, diagnostic tools, and disease severity.[26] Based on cause and disease severity, the 1-, 5-, and 10-year cumulative incidence of HE among cirrhotic patients ranges between 0% to 21%, 5% to 25%, and 7% to 42%, respectively. Within 2 years post-TIPS, the incidence of HE is between 20% and 55%. The prevalence estimates of MHE, HE in decompensated cirrhosis, and HE post-TIPS are 20% to 80%, 16% to 21%, and 10% to 50%, respectively.

In cirrhosis, major risk factors for overt HE include MHE, prior history of overt HE, sarcopenia, hyponatremia, epilepsy, T2DM, higher creatinine levels, higher bilirubin levels, lower levels of albumin, PPI use, nonselective beta-blockers use, and statin use. Risk factors for HE occurrence post-TIPS are older age, higher Child-Pugh score, higher MELD score, prior history of HE pre-TIPS, low PPG, and PPI use. The development of HE is associated with poor survival in cirrhotic patients. Factors associated with increased risk of mortality in HE include older age, high bilirubin levels, increase in creatinine levels, HE grade (III–IV vs I–II), PPI use, prior history of HE, MHE, and higher MELD score. Although combination therapy of rifaximin and lactulose is the AASLD/EASL-recommended treatment for the prevention of overt HE reoccurrence in cirrhosis, there is no evidence to support the use of either drug as prophylactic agents for HE reoccurrence prevention post-TIPS.

REFERENCES

1. Prakash R, Mullen KD. Mechanisms, diagnosis and management of hepatic encephalopathy. Nat Rev Gastroenterol Hepatol 2010;7(9):515.
2. Wijdicks EF. Hepatic encephalopathy. N Engl J Med 2016;375(17):1660–70.
3. Bajaj JS, Schubert CM, Heuman DM, et al. Persistence of cognitive impairment after resolution of overt hepatic encephalopathy. Gastroenterology 2010;138(7): 2332–40.

4. Campagna F, Montagnese S, Schiff S, et al. Cognitive impairment and electroencephalographic alterations before and after liver transplantation: what is reversible? Liver Transpl 2014;20(8):977–86.
5. Montagnese S, Bajaj JS. Impact of hepatic encephalopathy in cirrhosis on quality-of-life issues. Drugs 2019;79:11–6.
6. Umapathy S, Dhiman RK, Grover S, et al. Persistence of cognitive impairment after resolution of overt hepatic encephalopathy. Am J Gastroenterol 2014;109(7): 1011.
7. Vilstrup H, Amodio P, Bajaj J, et al. Hepatic encephalopathy in chronic liver disease: 2014 practice guideline by the European Association for the Study of the Liver and the American Association for the Study of Liver Diseases. J Hepatol 2014;61(3):642–59.
8. Bajaj JS, Wade JB, Gibson DP, et al. The multi-dimensional burden of cirrhosis and hepatic encephalopathy on patients and caregivers. Am J Gastroenterol 2011;106:1646–53.
9. Neff G III, Zachry W. Systematic review of the economic burden of overt hepatic encephalopathy and pharmacoeconomic impact of rifaximin. Pharmacoeconomics 2018;36(7):809–22.
10. Mellinger JL, Shedden K, Winder GS, et al. The high burden of alcoholic cirrhosis in privately insured persons in the United States. Hepatology 2018;68(3):872–82.
11. Butterworth RF. Pathogenesis of hepatic encephalopathy and brain edema in acute liver failure. J Clin Exp Hepatol 2015;5:S96–103.
12. Patel D, McPhail MJ, Cobbold JF, et al. Hepatic encephalopathy. Br J Hosp Med (Lond) 2012;73(2):79–85.
13. Lee WM, Larson AM, Stravitz RT. AASLD position paper: the management of acute liver failure: update 2011. Hepatology 2011;55(55):965–7.
14. Amodio P. Current diagnosis and classification of hepatic encephalopathy. J Clin Exp Hepatol 2018;8(4):432–7.
15. Elwir S, Rahimi RS. Hepatic encephalopathy: an update on the pathophysiology and therapeutic options. J Clin Transl Hepatol 2017;5(2):142.
16. Patidar KR, Bajaj JS. Neurologic consequences of liver disease. In: Sanyal AJ, Terrault N, editors. Zakim and Boyer's hepatology: a textbook of liver disease. Elsevier; 2018. p. 203.
17. Acharya C, Bajaj JS. Definition and changes in nomenclature of hepatic encephalopathy. In: Bajaj JS, editor. Diagnosis and management of hepatic encephalopathy: A Case-based Guide. Springer; 2018. p. 1–13.
18. Ferenci P, Lockwood A, Mullen K, et al. Hepatic encephalopathy—definition, nomenclature, diagnosis, and quantification: final report of the working party at the 11th World Congresses of Gastroenterology, Vienna, 1998. Hepatology 2002;35(3):716–21.
19. Amodio P. Hepatic encephalopathy: diagnosis and management. Liver Int 2018; 38(6):966–75.
20. Cordoba J, Ventura-Cots M, Simón-Talero M, et al. Characteristics, risk factors, and mortality of cirrhotic patients hospitalized for hepatic encephalopathy with and without acute-on-chronic liver failure (ACLF). J Hepatol 2014;60(2):275–81.
21. Romero-Gómez M, Montagnese S, Jalan R. Hepatic encephalopathy in patients with acute decompensation of cirrhosis and acute-on-chronic liver failure. J Hepatol 2015;62(2):437–47.
22. Montagnese S, Russo FP, Amodio P, et al. Hepatic encephalopathy 2018: a clinical practice guideline by the Italian Association for the Study of the Liver (AISF). Dig Liver Dis 2019;51(2):190–205.

23. Dharel N, Bajaj JS. Definition and nomenclature of hepatic encephalopathy. J Clin Exp Hepatol 2015;5:S37–41.
24. Amodio P, Montagnese S, Gatta A, et al. Characteristics of minimal hepatic encephalopathy. Metab Brain Dis 2004;19(3–4):253–67.
25. Poordad FF. Review article: the burden of hepatic encephalopathy. Aliment Pharmacol Ther 2007;25(SUPPL. 1):3–9.
26. Stepanova M, Mishra A, Venkatesan C, et al. In-hospital mortality and economic burden associated with hepatic encephalopathy in the United States from 2005 to 2009. Clin Gastroenterol Hepatol 2012;10(9):1034–41.e1.
27. Tapper EB, Henderson J, Baki J, et al. Incidence and predictors of hepatic encephalopathy in a population-based cohort of older Americans with cirrhosis: role of opiates, benzodiazepines and proton-pump inhibitors (PPIs). Hepatology 2018;68:138A.
28. Watson H, Jepsen P, Wong F, et al. Satavaptan treatment for ascites in patients with cirrhosis: a meta-analysis of effect on hepatic encephalopathy development. Metab Brain Dis 2013;28(2):301–5.
29. Ruiz-Margáin A, Macías-Rodríguez RU, Ampuero J, et al. Low phase angle is associated with the development of hepatic encephalopathy in patients with cirrhosis. World J Gastroenterol 2016;22(45):10064.
30. Goyal O, Sidhu S, Kishore H. Incidence, prevalence and natural history of minimal hepatic encephalopathy in cirrhosis. J Hepatol 2016;64(2):S279.
31. Hartmann IJ, Groeneweg M, Quero JC, et al. The prognostic significance of subclinical hepatic encephalopathy. Am J Gastroenterol 2000;95(8):2029–34.
32. Nilsson E, Anderson H, Sargenti K, et al. Clinical course and mortality by etiology of liver cirrhosis in Sweden: a population based, long-term follow-up study of 1317 patients. Aliment Pharmacol Ther 2019;49(11):1421–30.
33. Benvegnu L, Gios M, Boccato S, et al. Natural history of compensated viral cirrhosis: a prospective study on the incidence and hierarchy of major complications. Gut 2004;53(5):744–9.
34. Gentilini P, Laffi G, La Villa G, et al. Long course and prognostic factors of virus-induced cirrhosis of the liver. Am J Gastroenterol 1997;92(1):66–72.
35. Rowley MW, Choi M, Chen S, et al. Refractory hepatic encephalopathy after elective transjugular intrahepatic portosystemic shunt: risk factors and outcomes with revision. Cardiovasc Intervent Radiol 2018;41(11):1765–72.
36. Casadaban LC, Parvinian A, Minocha J, et al. Clearing the confusion over hepatic encephalopathy after TIPS creation: incidence, prognostic factors, and clinical outcomes. Dig Dis Sci 2015;60(4):1059–66.
37. Peter P, Andrej Z, Katarína ŠP, et al. Hepatic encephalopathy after transjugular intrahepatic portosystemic shunt in patients with recurrent variceal hemorrhage. Gastroenterol Res Pract 2013;2013:398172.
38. Nardelli S, Gioia S, Pasquale C, et al. Cognitive impairment predicts the occurrence of hepatic encephalopathy after transjugular intrahepatic portosystemic shunt. Am J Gastroenterol 2016;111(4):523.
39. Riggio O, Angeloni S, Salvatori FM, et al. Incidence, natural history, and risk factors of hepatic encephalopathy after transjugular intrahepatic portosystemic shunt with polytetrafluoroethylene-covered stent grafts. Am J Gastroenterol 2008;103(11):2738.
40. Schepis F, Vizzutti F, Garcia-Tsao G, et al. Under-dilated TIPS associate with efficacy and reduced encephalopathy in a prospective, non-randomized study of patients with cirrhosis. Clin Gastroenterol Hepatol 2018;16(7):1153–62.e7.

41. Song T, Rössle M, He F, et al. Transjugular intrahepatic portosystemic shunt for hepatorenal syndrome: a systematic review and meta-analysis. Dig Liver Dis 2018;50(4):323–30.
42. Das A, Dhiman RK, Saraswat VA, et al. Prevalence and natural history of subclinical hepatic encephalopathy in cirrhosis. J Gastroenterol Hepatol 2001;16(5): 531–5.
43. Groeneweg M, Moerland W, Quero JC, et al. Screening of subclinical hepatic encephalopathy. J Hepatol 2000;32(5):748–53.
44. Pomier-Layrargues G, Nguyen NH, Faucher C, et al. Subclinical hepatic encephalopathy in cirrhotic patients: prevalence and relationship to liver function. Can J Gastroenterol Hepatol 1991;5(4):121–5.
45. Rikkers L, Jenko P, Rudman D, et al. Subclinical hepatic encephalopathy: detection, prevalence, and relationship to nitrogen metabolism. Gastroenterology 1978;75(3):462–9.
46. Romero-Gómez M, Boza F, García-Valdecasas MS, et al. Subclinical hepatic encephalopathy predicts the development of overt hepatic encephalopathy. Am J Gastroenterol 2001;96(9):2718–23.
47. Sharma P, Sharma B, Puri V, et al. Critical flicker frequency: diagnostic tool for minimal hepatic encephalopathy. J Hepatol 2007;47(1):67–73.
48. Kircheis G, Wettstein M, Timmermann L, et al. Critical flicker frequency for quantification of low-grade hepatic encephalopathy. Hepatology 2002;35(2):357–66.
49. Wang A-J, Peng A-P, Li B-M, et al. Natural history of covert hepatic encephalopathy: an observational study of 366 cirrhotic patients. World J Gastroenterol 2017; 23(34):6321.
50. D'amico G, Morabito A, Pagliaro L, et al. Survival and prognostic indicators in compensated and decompensated cirrhosis. Dig Dis Sci 1986;31(5):468–75.
51. Jepsen P, Ott P, Andersen PK, et al. Clinical course of alcoholic liver cirrhosis: a Danish population-based cohort study. Hepatology 2010;51(5):1675–82.
52. Dooley JS, Lok AS, Garcia-Tsao G, et al. Sherlock's diseases of the liver and biliary system. Hoboken (NJ): John Wiley & Sons; 2018.
53. Nolte W, Wiltfang J, Schindler C, et al. Portosystemic hepatic encephalopathy after transjugular intrahepatic portosystemic shunt in patients with cirrhosis: clinical, laboratory, psychometric, and electroencephalographic investigations. Hepatology 1998;28(5):1215–25.
54. Amodio P, Del Piccolo F, Pettenò E, et al. Prevalence and prognostic value of quantified electroencephalogram (EEG) alterations in cirrhotic patients. J Hepatol 2001;35(1):37–45.
55. Papatheodoridis GV, Goulis J, Leandro G, et al. Transjugular intrahepatic portosystemic shunt compared with endoscopic treatment for prevention of variceal rebleeding: a meta-analysis. Hepatology 1999;30(3):612–22.
56. Somberg KA, Riegler JL, LaBerge JM, et al. Hepatic encephalopathy after transjugular intrahepatic portosystemic shunts: incidence and risk factors. Am J Gastroenterol 1995;90(4):549–55.
57. Bai M, Qi X, Yang Z, et al. Predictors of hepatic encephalopathy after transjugular intrahepatic portosystemic shunt in cirrhotic patients: a systematic review. J Gastroenterol Hepatol 2011;26(6):943–51.
58. Fonio P, Discalzi A, Calandri M, et al. Incidence of hepatic encephalopathy after transjugular intrahepatic portosystemic shunt (TIPS) according to its severity and temporal grading classification. Radiol Med 2017;122(9):713–21.
59. Lewis DS, Lee TH, Konanur M, et al. Proton pump inhibitor use is associated with an increased frequency of new or worsening hepatic encephalopathy after

transjugular intrahepatic portosystemic shunt creation. J Vasc Interv Radiol 2019; 30(2):163–9.

60. Nardelli S, Lattanzi B, Torrisi S, et al. Sarcopenia is risk factor for development of hepatic encephalopathy after transjugular intrahepatic portosystemic shunt placement. Clin Gastroenterol Hepatol 2017;15(6):934–6.

61. Yao J, Zuo L, An G, et al. Risk factors for hepatic encephalopathy after transjugular intrahepatic portosystemic shunt in patients with hepatocellular carcinoma and portal hypertension. J Gastrointestin Liver Dis 2015;24(3):301–7.

62. Rowley MW, Choi M, Chen S, et al. Race and gradient difference are associated with increased risk of hepatic encephalopathy hospital admission after transjugular intrahepatic portosystemic shunt placement. J Clin Exp Hepatol 2018;8(3): 256–61.

63. Riggio O, Nardelli S, Moscucci F, et al. Hepatic encephalopathy after transjugular intrahepatic portosystemic shunt. Clin Liver Dis 2012;16(1):133–46.

64. Sturm L, Bettinger D, Giesler M, et al. Treatment with proton pump inhibitors increases the risk for development of hepatic encephalopathy after implantation of transjugular intrahepatic portosystemic shunt (TIPS). United European Gastroenterol J 2018;6(9):1380–90.

65. Berlioux P, Robic MA, Poirson H, et al. Pre-transjugular intrahepatic portosystemic shunts (TIPS) prediction of post-TIPS overt hepatic encephalopathy: the critical flicker frequency is more accurate than psychometric tests. Hepatology 2014;59(2):622–9.

66. Casado M, Bosch J, García-Pagán JC, et al. Clinical events after transjugular intrahepatic portosystemic shunt: correlation with hemodynamic findings. Gastroenterology 1998;114(6):1296–303.

67. Riggio O, Merlli M, Pedretti G, et al. Hepatic encephalopathy after transjugular intrahepatic portosystemic shunt. Incidence and risk factors. Dig Dis Sci 1996; 41(3):578–84.

68. Weissenborn K. Hepatic encephalopathy: definition, clinical grading and diagnostic principles. Drugs 2019;79(s1):5–9.

69. Weissenborn K. Challenges in diagnosing hepatic encephalopathy. Neurochem Res 2014;40(2):265–73.

70. Ampuero J, Montoliú C, Simón-Talero M, et al. Minimal hepatic encephalopathy identifies patients at risk of faster cirrhosis progression. J Gastroenterol Hepatol 2018;33(3):718–25.

71. Bannister CA, Orr JG, Reynolds AV, et al. Natural history of patients taking Rifaximin-alpha for recurrent hepatic encephalopathy and risk of future overt episodes and mortality: a post-hoc analysis of clinical trials data. Clin Ther 2016; 38(5):1081–9.

72. Chang KV, Chen JD, Wu WT, et al. Is sarcopenia associated with hepatic encephalopathy in liver cirrhosis? A systematic review and meta-analysis. J Formos Med Assoc 2019;118(4):833–42.

73. Dam G, Vilstrup H, Watson H, et al. Proton pump inhibitors as a risk factor for hepatic encephalopathy and spontaneous bacterial peritonitis in patients with cirrhosis with ascites. Hepatology 2016;64(4):1265–72.

74. Guevara M, Baccaro ME, Ríos J, et al. Risk factors for hepatic encephalopathy in patients with cirrhosis and refractory ascites: relevance of serum sodium concentration. Liver Int 2010;30(8):1137–42.

75. Guevara M, Baccaro ME, Torre A, et al. Hyponatremia is a risk factor of hepatic encephalopathy in patients with cirrhosis: a prospective study with time-dependent analysis. Am J Gastroenterol 2009;104(6):1382–9.

76. Jepsen P, Christensen J, Weissenborn K, et al. Epilepsy as a risk factor for hepatic encephalopathy in patients with cirrhosis: a cohort study. BMC Gastroenterol 2016;16(1):1–6.

77. Jepsen P, Watson H, Andersen PK, et al. Diabetes as a risk factor for hepatic encephalopathy in cirrhosis patients. J Hepatol 2015;63(5):1133–8.

78. Riggio O, Amodio P, Farcomeni A, et al. A model for predicting development of overt hepatic encephalopathy in patients with cirrhosis. Clin Gastroenterol Hepatol 2015;13(7):1346–52.

79. Tapper EB, Parikh ND, Sengupta N, et al. A risk score to predict the development of hepatic encephalopathy in a population-based cohort of patients with cirrhosis. Hepatology 2018;68(4):1498–507.

80. Sigal SH, Stanca CM, Kontorinis N, et al. Diabetes mellitus is associated with hepatic encephalopathy in patients with HCV cirrhosis. Am J Gastroenterol 2006; 101(7):1490.

81. Nardone R, Taylor AC, Höller Y, et al. Minimal hepatic encephalopathy: a review. Neurosci Res 2016;111:1–12.

82. Nardelli S, Gioia S, Ridola L, et al. Proton pump inhibitors are associated with minimal and overt hepatic encephalopathy and increased mortality in patients with cirrhosis. Hepatology 2019;70(2):640–9.

83. Sharma BC, Sharma P, Agrawal A, et al. Secondary prophylaxis of hepatic encephalopathy: an open-label randomized controlled trial of lactulose versus placebo. Gastroenterology 2009;137(3):885–91.e1.

84. Bustamante J, Rimola A, Ventura P-J, et al. Prognostic significance of hepatic encephalopathy in patients with cirrhosis. J Hepatol 1999;30(5):890–5.

85. Stewart CA, Malinchoc M, Kim WR, et al. Hepatic encephalopathy as a predictor of survival in patients with end-stage liver disease. Liver Transpl 2007;13(10): 1366–71.

86. D'Amico G, Garcia-Tsao G, Pagliaro L. Natural history and prognostic indicators of survival in cirrhosis: a systematic review of 118 studies. J Hepatol 2006;44(1): 217–31.

87. Wong RJ, Gish RG, Ahmed A. Hepatic encephalopathy is associated with significantly increased mortality among patients awaiting liver transplantation. Liver Transpl 2014;20(12):1454–61.

88. Ampuero J, Simón M, Montoliú C, et al. Minimal hepatic encephalopathy and critical flicker frequency are associated with survival of patients with cirrhosis. Gastroenterology 2015;149(6):1483–9.

89. Patidar KR, Thacker LR, Wade JB, et al. Covert hepatic encephalopathy is independently associated with poor survival and increased risk of hospitalization. Am J Gastroenterol 2014;109(11):1757.

90. Berry K, Lerrigo R, Liou IW, et al. Association between transjugular intrahepatic portosystemic shunt and survival in patients with cirrhosis. Clin Gastroenterol Hepatol 2016;14(1):118–23.

91. Jalan R, Elton RA, Redhead DN, et al. Analysis of prognostic variables in the prediction of mortality, shunt failure, variceal rebleeding and encephalopathy following the transjugular intrahepatic portosystemic stent-shunt for variceal haemorrhage. J Hepatol 1995;23(2):123–8.

92. Vilstrup H, Amodio P, Bajaj J, et al. Hepatic encephalopathy in chronic liver disease: 2014 practice guideline by the American Association for the Study of Liver Diseases and the European Association for the Study of the Liver. Hepatology 2014;60(2):715–35.

93. Gluud LL, Vilstrup H, Morgan MY. Non-absorbable disaccharides versus placebo/no intervention and lactulose versus lactitol for the prevention and treatment of hepatic encephalopathy in people with cirrhosis. Cochrane Database Syst Rev 2016;(5):CD003044.
94. Bass NM, Mullen KD, Sanyal A, et al. Rifaximin treatment in hepatic encephalopathy. N Engl J Med 2010;362(12):1071–81.

Pathophysiology of Hepatic Encephalopathy

Ariel Jaffe, MD[a], Joseph K. Lim, MD[a,b], Sofia Simona Jakab, MD[a,b,*]

KEYWORDS

- Liver cirrhosis • Hepatic encephalopathy • Ammonia • Neurotoxicity • TNF-Alpha
- Gut-liver-brain axis • Neurotransmitters • Cannabinoids

KEY POINTS

- Ammonia remains central to the pathophysiology of hepatic encephalopathy (HE), and various HE precipitants affect ammonia production, excretion, and neurotoxicity.
- New mechanisms related to inflammation, gut microbiome, and neurotransmitters have been identified.
- In addition to the liver and brain, other organs such as the gut, kidneys, and muscle are critical for the metabolism of ammonia and glutamine, the key molecules in HE pathophysiology.
- Better understanding of the intricate pathophysiologic mechanisms of HE is paramount for a comprehensive approach to the management of HE.

INTRODUCTION

Hepatic encephalopathy (HE) represents a spectrum of reversible neuropsychiatric changes that are driven by a variety of underlying pathogenic mechanisms. These symptoms range from mild cognitive disturbances to ataxia and even coma. HE is a significant source of morbidity among patients with both acute and chronic liver disease as well as patients with high degrees of portosystemic shunting. There has been a continuous increase in cirrhosis in the United States, and up to 60% of these patients will develop some degree of HE. Also, HE is the most common reason for hospitalization in patients with decompensated cirrhosis, accounting for more than 100,000 annual admissions with total hospital charges of 7 billion dollars[1] and increased mortality.[2] In addition, there is significant family/caregiver burden given the need for high-level supportive care, with depression and anxiety reported in up to 20% of caregivers.[3]

[a] Section of Digestive Diseases, Yale Liver Center, Yale University School of Medicine, 333 Cedar Street, LMP 1080, New Haven, CT 06520-8019, USA; [b] VA Connecticut Healthcare System, West Haven, Connecticut, USA
* Corresponding author.
E-mail address: simona.jakab@yale.edu

Clin Liver Dis 24 (2020) 175–188
https://doi.org/10.1016/j.cld.2020.01.002
1089-3261/20/Published by Elsevier Inc.

Understanding the underlying pathophysiology of HE is of critical importance in order to optimally manage this condition. Although neurotoxicity secondary to hyperammonemia remains central to the development of hepatic encephalopathy, in the last decade multiple new pathogenetic mechanisms have been identified.

HEPATIC ENCEPHALOPATHY PRECIPITANTS

Ammonia is a small nitrogenous metabolite that originates from the degradation of proteins and amino acids. Most of the research on the underlying pathophysiology of HE has been focused on the buildup of this nitrogenous waste product in the blood and brain of humans. Although hyperammonemia is not the only mechanism in the development of HE, substantial research has proved that it plays a significant role and has multiple devastating cellular effects.

There are a variety of HE precipitants that act through one or more of the 3 major pathways related to ammonia metabolism and toxicity: increased production, impaired excretion, and increased neurotoxicity (**Table 1**). Identifying and correcting the precipitating factor is the cornerstone of clinical management of HE. The most common precipitants of HE include infections, gastrointestinal bleeding, intravascular hypovolemia often secondary to diuretic overdosing, and constipation.[4] Understanding the complex intricacies of the pathogenetic mechanisms involved allows a comprehensive approach to the management of HE and helps clinicians target new pathways for the treatment of this condition.

AMMONIA PRODUCTION

The 2 main sites of ammonia production are the small/large intestine (50%) and the kidneys (40%).

Within the *intestine*, 2 mechanisms exist: (1) urea from dietary protein is broken down into ammonia and carbon dioxide exclusively via urease-producing bacteria (ie, Klebsiella, Proteus) predominantly in the large intestine, and (2) direct amino acid degradation of glutamine under the effect of the glutaminase in the enterocytes

Table 1 Pathophysiology of clinical precipitants of hepatic encephalopathy	
Pathophysiologic Pathway	**Precipitants**
Increased Ammonia Production	Gastrointestinal bleed Intravascular hypovolemia, overdiuresis Hypokalemia Acidosis Excessive protein intake Diabetes mellitus
Impaired Ammonia Excretion	Constipation Renal dysfunction Hypovolemia, overdiuresis Sarcopenia Portosystemic shunting Zinc deficiency Branched-chain amino acid deficiency
Increased Neurotoxicity	Infection Medications/substance abuse Hyponatremia Hyperglycemia

generates glutamate and free ammonia. This unionized form of ammonia can then cross the intestinal epithelium freely and enter the portal circulation. Ionization of ammonia depends on the colonic luminal pH, with a more acidic pH leading to protonation and trapping of ammonium (NH_4+) within the lumen. Of note, nonabsorbable disaccharides, such as lactulose, lower colonic pH in addition to their laxative effect and decrease ammonia reabsorption.

Although one of the major sources of ammonia is from *protein* breakdown by gut bacteria, low protein diets should be avoided in patients with hepatic encephalopathy. Randomized trials have shown that even during an acute episode of HE, regular protein versus low protein intake caused no difference in HE resolution.[5] Most importantly, protein malnutrition leads to sarcopenia, which is associated with higher mortality and increased risk of hepatic encephalopathy, given the important role the muscles play in nitrogen metabolism for patients with cirrhosis.[6] Plant-based proteins may offer additional benefits, as they contain less methionine and cysteine and more arginine and ornithine, which are metabolized as part of the urea cycle. Increased fiber intake also shortens bowel transit time and decreases ammonia absorption.[7]

Within the *kidneys*, the proximal tubular cells are capable of generating ammonia from glutamine and creating bicarbonate as a byproduct. Therefore, the renal production of ammonia is driven by the body's acid-base status and potassium balance. In the setting of metabolic acidosis or hypokalemia, glutamine is used to facilitate the disposal of acid or recovery of potassium. Through this mechanism, renal ammoniagenesis increases arterial ammonia levels.[8] In addition, intravascular hypovolemia in the setting of gastrointestinal bleeding and overdiuresis enhances renal ammonia production, mediated through angiotensin II,[9] whereas volume expansion either as volume challenge or just by stopping diuretics is beneficial for patients with worsening hepatic encephalopathy.[10]

Smaller contributors of ammonia production include release of ammonia from muscles via the adenylic acid metabolism, which plays a role in the purine nucleotide cycle, along with release of glutamine from senescent red blood cells.[11]

AMMONIA EXCRETION

The major site of ammonia catabolism is the *urea cycle* (Krebs-Henseleit cycle), which exclusively takes place within the liver. Through this mechanism, 2 molecules of ammonia and one molecule of carbon dioxide generate urea and water. Urea is easily able to cross membranes given its small size and therefore is able to enter back into the intestines and the kidneys for excretion.

The ammonia concentration within the portal vein is 5 to 10x higher than that of the systemic circulation.[11] When there is reduced capability of the liver to detoxify ammonia, due to either hepatocellular damage or shunting around the liver from portal hypertension or spontaneous/iatrogenic portosystemic shunts, there is resultant buildup within the systemic circulation.

The kidneys contribute to ammonia excretion through parallel H+ and ammonia secretion in the collecting duct, generating *ammonium*, which is eliminated through urine. Of note, almost all urinary ammonia is from renal ammoniagenesis. The proportion of ammonia generated that is excreted in the urine depends on several factors, most importantly acid-base and potassium balance, protein intake, and glucocorticoid hormones, but overall renal venous ammonia exceeds arterial ammonia, meaning that the kidneys actually increase systemic ammonia.[12] In the normal physiologic state, about 50% of ammonia gets excreted in the urine with the remainder being returned to the systemic circulation via the renal vein. In acidosis, the kidneys excrete hydrogen ions in the urine and convert ammonia to ammonium. In alkalosis, there is significant reduction in renal excretion of ammonia; similarly, when the renal perfusion is reduced (such as in dehydration and overdiuresis) there is a reduction in ammonia excretion.[11]

Muscles are capable of temporarily detoxifying ammonia by converting ammonia into *glutamine* via glutamine synthetase (GS). Impaired hepatic clearance of ammonia upregulates the gene coding for GS,[13] and skeletal muscles become a significant site of ammonia metabolism for patients with cirrhosis. Therefore, sarcopenia is a risk factor for HE,[14] and improving muscle mass is beneficial for HE treatment.

Studies have shown an abnormal ratio in *branched-chain amino acids* (BCAAs), including isoleucine, leucine, and valine along with aromatic amino acids in patients with cirrhosis, thought to be secondary to increased metabolism within skeletal muscles.[15] Given the role of BCAAs to generate glutamate, BCAA deficiency leads to a reduced ability of the skeletal muscles to convert ammonia to glutamine. A recent review of 16 randomized controlled trials (RCTs) showed that BCAA supplementation had a beneficial effect on HE, with a number needed to treat of 5.[16] American Association for the Study of Liver Diseases recommends BCAAs as an alternative or additional agent to treat patients who are not responsive to conventional therapy.[4]

Therapeutic strategies focused on enhancing these catabolic pathways have been evaluated for patients with HE. *L-Ornithine L-Aspartate* (LOLA) increases both ureagenesis and glutamine synthesis: L-ornithine serves as an intermediary in the urea cycle in periportal hepatocytes in the liver and as an activator of carbamoyl phosphate synthetase and, as L-aspartate, by transamination to glutamate via GS in perivenous hepatocytes as well as by skeletal muscle and brain. Intravenous LOLA improved psychometric testing and postprandial venous ammonia levels in patients with persistent HE.[17]

Ammonia scavengers used for treatment of inborn errors of the urea cycle may also have therapeutic potential in HE treatment. Their mechanism of action targets primarily glutamine excretion. For ornithine phenylacetate, the L-ornithine component acts as a substrate for the synthesis of glutamine from ammonia and glutamate in skeletal muscle, and the phenylacetate component combines with glutamine to form phenylacetylglutamine, which is then excreted by the kidneys. Glycerol phenylbutyrate conjugates with glutamine in the liver and kidneys, forming a compound excreted in the urine.[18,19]

Although inherited urea cycle disorders are very rare, patients with HE who do not respond to the usual treatment, especially if their liver dysfunction and/or portosystemic shunting are discordant with their HE severity or refractoriness, may need further evaluation in this regard and treatment adjustment using ammonia scavengers.

An important microelement for pathogenesis of HE is *zinc* (Zn), which is a cofactor in the urea cycle and therefore critical in ammonia detoxification. Prevalence of Zn deficiency is very high in cirrhosis, with recent studies showing more than 90% of patients affected.[20] A meta-analysis showed that Zn supplementation can improve some psychometric tests.[21]

AMMONIA NEUROTOXICITY

Under physiologic conditions, most of the ammonia is in the weak acidic NH_4+ form. It has been shown that this ion has an almost identical ionic radius and diffusion coefficient to potassium ($K+$) and can therefore compete and bind to various $K+$ channels and transporters.[22] Ammonia is therefore able to cross the blood-brain-barrier both by passive diffusion in the uncharged ammonia form, as well as through active transport through various ion transporters in its NH4+ form. Some evidence also exists that transportation occurs via specific mammalian ammonia transporter as well as through special aquaporin channels (specifically aquaporin-8).[23,24]

ASTROCYTE CELL DYSFUNCTION SECONDARY TO AMMONIA AND GLUTAMINE: OSMOTIC GLIOPATHY, OXIDATIVE STRESS, MICROGLIAL CELL ACTIVATION

Ammonia preferentially enters the astrocytes, as these cells have the highest affinity for potassium and are also the only brain cells that contain GS, allowing for the detoxification of ammonia through generation of glutamine. In fact, GS has a higher affinity for ammonia than it does for glutamate in astrocytes, and these cells are likely to take up to 4 times as much ammonia than any other cell type. Ammonia acts both as a substrate and as a product for a variety of biochemical reactions and is therefore capable of causing multiple cellular changes that alter cellular function; these changes range from altering pH, membrane potentials, and electrolyte balance, to impairing oxidative metabolism via inhibition of the rate-limiting enzyme in the tricarboxylic acid cycle, altering calcium signaling, activating mitochondrial permeability transition leading to cell dysfunction, and changing neurotransmitter equilibrium potentials.[25]

A variety of studies have demonstrated low-grade cerebral edema in cirrhotic patients via indirect measurements of water content using MRI.[26,27] There are 2 mechanisms that contribute to cerebral edema in liver disease. Glutamine itself acts as an osmole, and increased intracellular concentrations of this molecule within astrocytes develop as these cells try and detoxify ammonia using GS. This creates an osmolar gradient resulting in astrocyte swelling and what is known as an osmotic gliopathy.[11] Secondarily, glutamine enters mitochondria where special glutaminases catabolize it back into ammonia. This mitochondrial ammonia accumulation results in generation of reactive oxygen species resulting in increased mitochondrial permeability and ultimately leads to astrocyte cell dysfunction and swelling.[28]

In chronic liver disease there is only mild astrocyte swelling, but it ultimately results in oxidative stress and cell dysfunction, whereas in acute liver failure there is significant astrocyte swelling with increase in intracranial pressure and most fatally cerebral herniation. Recent literature has also shown persistent deficits in working memory, response inhibition, and learning capacity after resolutions of overt HE, which was suggested to be due to astrocyte senescence. These studies found that ammonia inhibits astrocyte proliferation and that post mortem patients with HE had increased messenger RNA levels of senescence-associated gene.[29]

Factors that cause astrocyte swelling aside from hyperammonemia include hyponatremia, which is a common finding in cirrhotic patients. The primary mechanism is due to hypersecretion of antidiuretic hormone, prompted by a low effective arterial volume secondary to splanchnic vasodilation. Hyponatremia is associated with reduced concentration of organic osmolytes in the brain, making it more susceptible to cellular damage in times of either increased intracellular osmolality or hypoosmolar extracellular environments.[30] Hyponatremia therefore remains as a potential second osmotic hit to astrocytes, and correction of this electrolyte disturbance is important for prevention/treatment of HE.

In addition to astrocyte cell dysfunction, neuropathology studies haven noted microglial cell activation,[31] which results in a proinflammatory state leading to monocyte recruitment as well as increased cytokine gene expression within the brain.[32] Using PET imaging to localize activated microglial cell proteins (ie, mitochondrial translator protein), increased signal intensity has been noted in the anterior cingulate cortex, which is a structure associated with the control of attention.[33] Neuronal cell damage and death are also well documented and can result in acquired (non-Wilsonian) hepatocerebral degeneration, postshunt myelopathy, and direct cerebellar damage.[34] In addition, liver failures can contribute to neuronal death in Wernicke encephalopathy, as the liver is the main site of thiamine synthesis and storage.[34] This underscores the important need to supplement thiamine in patients with end-stage liver disease. The mechanisms underlying neuronal damage are similar to the aforementioned pathways and include N-methyl-D-aspartate (NMDA) receptor–mediated excitotoxicity, lactic acidosis, oxidative stress, and presence of proinflammatory cytokines.[34]

Despite the role of ammonia in the development of HE, other important factors exist, as patients can have elevated arterial ammonia levels without signs or symptoms of HE. Similarly, patients with normal ammonia levels can have signs of HE in acute and chronic liver failure, and the degree of hyperammonemia does not always correlate well with severity of HE.[35] Major contributors to HE include a variety of other neurotoxins, nutritional deficiencies/metabolic abnormalities, systemic and central inflammation, and changes in specific neurotransmission, specifically activation of GABA.

TUMOR NECROSIS FACTOR ALPHA THEORY: SYSTEMIC AND CENTRAL INFLAMMATION

Systemic inflammation is a major mechanism behind the development of HE. A variety of different inciting events can exacerbate the inflammatory status of cirrhotic patients, whom at baseline have been shown to have higher levels of tumor necrosis factor (TNF) alpha than noncirrhotic patients.[36] The most common triggers include infection or direct hepatocellular injury, which would release proinflammatory cytokines such as TNF-alpha, interleukin (IL)-1B, and IL-6. Multiple studies have demonstrated the synergistic relationship between systemic inflammation and ammonia-induced cerebral dysfunction.[37,38]

Several sources lead to increased TNF-alpha levels in patients with liver disease. One major source results from gut flora translocation. Because of bacterial overgrowth, bowel dysmotility, bowel vascular congestion, and edema, common in patients with liver disease, there is increased bacterial translocation compared with healthy patients.[39] In addition, advanced liver disease causes impaired ability of the reticuloendothelial system to destroy translocated bacteria within the portal circulation (either due to impaired function or due to increased shunting), and resultant endotoxemia from gram-negative bacteria develops.[40]

Other factors that increase the risk of bacterial translocation include the use of *proton pump inhibitors* (PPIs), as reduced stomach acidity can lead to intestinal bacterial overgrowth and increased risk of bacterial translocation. Studies have found up to 78% of cirrhotic patients to be on PPI therapy, with greater than 50% on therapy for inappropriate clinical reasons.[41] One study looking at the data from 3 RCTs of patients with cirrhosis and ascites found an increased risk of developing both HE and spontaneous bacterial peritonitis with the use of a PPI.[42] Another case-control study by Tsai and colleagues[43] evaluating 1166 patients with cirrhosis and HE found that use of PPIs increased the risk of HE, with a dose-dependent effect. This should caution clinicians to do a thorough medication review and consider discontinuation of PPI if there is no significant clinical indication or benefit.

Endotoxins from gram-negative bacteria result in the release of TNF-alpha from the monocyte/macrophage system. Levels of TNF-alpha have been shown to be associated with the presence of HE and the severity of HE, regardless of the precipitating event.[44] In another study, patients with cirrhosis, but without overt HE, were given amino acid solution resulting in hyperammonemia. HE developed only in those patients who had concurrent systemic inflammatory response syndrome, suggesting the role of TNF-alpha as a critical factor in the neuropsychological effects from ammonia.[38] Multiple studies have shown that TNF-alpha alters neurotransmission, via inhibition of astrocyte uptake of glutamate along with enhancement of glutamate receptor–mediated neurotoxicity.[45] In addition, cerebrovascular endothelial cells exposed to TNF-alpha have an increased capacity for ammonia transport, further potentiating its toxic effects on central nervous system (CNS) effects.[46] Finally, TNF can directly cause cerebral edema by increasing microvascular permeability, causing capillary fluid leakage.[47] Of note, common known precipitants of HE such as infection and gastrointestinal bleeding cause significant increase in TNF-alpha production,[48] suggesting the clinical importance of this pathophysiologic pathway.

GUT-LIVER-BRAIN AXIS: GUT MICROBIOTA

Changes in the gut flora have been shown to play a major role in the development of HE. Studies have shown that decreased production of bile acids secondary to end-stage liver disease results in increased proliferation of more pathogenic, urease-producing bacteria such as Enterobacteriaceae with resultant reduction in protective commensal bacteria such as Lachnospiraceae.[49] The importance of gut flora and gut-liver-brain axis in HE was studied by Ahluwalia and colleagues,[50] who evaluated varying effects of specific gut bacterial taxa in 187 patients. They found that patients with HE had more systemic inflammation, dysbiosis, and hyperammonemia compared with controls or patients with cirrhosis without HE. In addition, specific gut microbial changes were linked with levels of systemic inflammation, ammonia, and neuronal/astrocytic dysfunction as measured with multi-modal MRI.[50] Another study by Bajaj and colleagues[51] compared the gut microbiome of cirrhotic patients with and without HE and found alterations not only in the microbiome (higher Enterobacteriaceae and Fusobacteriaceae species) but also in degrees of endotoxemia and systemic inflammation as measured by serum IL-6, TNF-alpha, IL-2, and IL-13. Based on this theory of gut flora/gut-liver-brain axis, the use of a variety of microbiome-altering medication has been tried. Probiotics are of particular interest, and a recent meta-analysis including 14 RCTs found it may reduce serum ammonia and endotoxin levels, improve HE, and prevent overt HE.[52] In addition, the use of fecal microbiota transplant has also been explored as a possible therapy. Bajaj and colleagues[53] recently published the results of the first randomized clinical trial of fecal microbiota transplant (FMT) in patients with cirrhosis and recurrent HE. They followed patients for more than 12 months and found that patients treated with FMT had less hospitalizations and HE episodes compared with the standard of care arm. In addition, there were no concerning long-term safety events. Larger studies involving FMT for treatment of recurrent HE are ongoing.

NEUROTRANSMITTERS AND MINERALS

Alterations in several neurotransmitters play a major role in the underlying pathophysiology of HE.

Glutamate

Glutamate is the main excitatory neurotransmitter in the brain, with reduced transmission occurring in HE. There are a variety of changes that occur within the glutamate system as a result of elevated ammonia within the CNS and include alterations in expression and activity of glutamate transporters in the synaptic cleft,[54] changes in synaptic transmission via reduced release of glutamate in the nerve terminals secondary to reduced synthesis from glutamine,[55] prevention of action potential invasion in the presynaptic terminal,[56] and reduced glutamate release by blockage of glutamate receptors.[57] These alterations contribute to the neurologic symptoms seen in HE. In addition, acute elevations of ammonia result in excessive NMDA receptor activation, which leads to significant neurotoxicity, although this finding is not seen with chronic hyperammonemia.[58]

Monoamines: Histamine and Serotonin

Another neurotransmitter system affected by ammonia is the monoamine system. It has been shown that activation of histaminergic systems contributes to certain symptoms including sleep cycle disturbances and alerted motor functions in HE. A variety of studies have found elevated histamine levels in plasma and brain tissue, and the mechanism is possibly due to increase in the brain neutral amino acid transporter system.[59]

Increased concentrations of 5-hydroxyindoleacetic acid (5-HIAA), a serotonin (5-HT) metabolite, have been found in children with urea cycle disorders and correlate with plasma ammonia levels.[60] In addition, CSF 5-HIAA levels have been found to be elevated in brain tissue from patients with cirrhosis who died in hepatic comas,[61] suggesting increased 5-HT turnover and metabolism in hyperammonemia. The mechanisms that result in increased 5-HT turnover include stimulation of precursor L-tryptophan uptake, increased monoamine oxidase A expression, and decreased storage/increased intracellular oxidation of 5-HT leading to decreased availability for release from presynaptic terminals.[62] These reduced levels are believed to contribute to the neuropsychiatric symptoms including depression and sleep pattern alterations.[63]

Gamma Aminobutyric Acid

Gamma aminobutyric acid (GABA) is the main inhibitory neurotransmitter in the brain, resulting in impaired motor function and consciousness.[36] Increased GABAergic transmission was first suggested as a contributor to HE when visual evoked response (VER) patterns in animals with HE were found to be identical to normal animals treated with GABA receptor complex activators.[64] It has also been shown that there is upregulation of the 18-kDa translator protein, which plays a role in the production of endogenous benzodiazepines (ie, neurosteroids) that modulate GABA type A receptors.[65] In addition, it has been shown that there are increased concentrations of the peripheral type benzodiazepine receptor in the mitochondrial membrane of astrocytes in response to ammonia exposure. This has been thought to alter energy metabolism leading to astrocyte swelling causing an Alzheimer type II histopathological appearance, as well as increase synthesis of neurosteroids via stimulation of cholesterol transport across the mitochondrial membrane.[25,58] Based on these observations, clinical studies using benzodiazepine site antagonists such as flumazenil have been conducted in patients with HE and have resulted in electroencephalogram and clinical improvement,[66] although these effects were only of short duration.

The underlying pathophysiology of this increased GABAergic tone is not completely elucidated, but it may be related to alterations in gene expression of GABA receptors, increase in brain content of GABA agonists, and/or increases in endogenous modulators such as benzodiazepines and neurosteroids.[67]

A recently studied neurosteroid, allopregnanolone, which works by activating GABA type A receptors, was found to be increased in brain tissue from patients with advanced HE (coma).[68] A new agent GR 3027, which is an antagonist of a neurosteroidsite, has shown promising results in improving symptoms in patients with HE.[69]

Manganese

Maganese (Mn) is an essential metal required for a variety of important physiologic functions, but it has been identified as an important neurotoxin related to end-stage liver disease. Mn uptake is tightly regulated, and any excess gets excreted into the bile. Chronic liver disease causes elevated Mn levels, which can accumulate and deposit in the CNS. The major site of Mn deposition is within the basal ganglia, and in particular the globuspallidus, as shown on brain MRI. This buildup leads to a variety of cellular disturbances, with particular susceptibility in astrocytes due to their high affinity and specific manganese transport system.[70] Once taken up by the astrocyte, Mn tends to sequester in the mitochondria leading to disruption of oxidative phosphorylation and cellular stress. In addition, Mn deposition leads to impaired glutamate transport leading to increased extracellular concentration as well as loss of postsynaptic dopamine-D2 binding with selective dopaminergic dysfunction causing impaired astrocyte-neuronal interactions.[70,71] The clinical consequence of Mn deposition is the development of extrapyramidal symptoms, with motor disturbances and neuropsychiatric and cognitive disabilities similar to Parkinson disease.[72] A recent study of 51 cirrhotic patients being evaluated for liver transplantation showed that up to 22% exhibited these symptoms.[73] Treatment with L-Dopa may result in clinical improvement, whereas liver transplantation caused resolution of these symptoms in some patients.[72]

OTHER CLINICALLY RELEVANT CONDITIONS AND PATHOPHYSIOLOGIC CORRELATES
Diabetes and Insulin Resistance

HE seems to be an associated with diabetes mellitus (DM) and insulin resistance. A recent study from Butt and colleagues[74] showed that patients admitted with decompensated cirrhosis were more likely to develop HE and have more severe HE on presentation if they had concurrent DM. Another study of cirrhotic patients with ascites assessed first-time occurrence of HE and also found DM to be a risk factor for development and severity of HE.[75] The underlying pathophysiology behind DM and HE correlation involves a variety of factors. Patients with DM have higher incidence of delayed gastric emptying, increased orocecal time, and intestinal bacterial overgrowth, which may play a role in increased intestinal ammonia production and bacterial translocation.[74] Other postulated mechanisms include increased glutaminase activity within the kidney, liver, and small intestine leading to increased ammonia production, excess proinflammatory cytokines (IL-6, TNF-alpha) leading to systemic inflammation, and reduced sensitivity to insulin resulting in increased muscle breakdown and protein catabolism.[76] Metformin was recently shown to reduce the risk of HE in diabetic cirrhotic patients by partial inhibition of glutaminase and improved insulin resistance.[77]

CANNABINOIDS

Data regarding cannabinoids and HE are more clinically relevant than ever, given increased use of cannabinoid products. An older study by Magen and colleagues[78] evaluated the therapeutic effects of cannabidiol (CBD), a nonpsychoactive constituent of Cannabis sativa, in mice with HE caused by bile duct ligation. The cognitive function in the 8-arm maze and the T-maze tests, as well as locomotor function in the open field test were impaired by the ligation and were improved by CBD. The investigators further explored possible underlying mechanisms, showing that the beneficial effects of CBD were secondary to a combination of antiinflammatory activity and activation of 5-HT(1A) receptor, leading to improvement of the neurologic deficits without affecting 5-HT(1A) receptor expression or liver function.[79]

A more recent study[79] evaluated the acute effect of cannabis on plasma, liver, and brain ammonia dynamics. Cannabis intake caused time- and route-dependent increases in plasma ammonia concentrations in human cannabis users, whereas in mice there was reduced brain GS activity and increased brain and plasma ammonia concentrations. Further studies are needed to determine the effectiveness and safety of nonprescription formulations of cannabis for patients with cirrhosis.

SUMMARY

The optimal treatment of HE is much more than lactulose. As we better understand the underlying complex pathophysiology of hepatic encephalopathy, clinicians have additional pathways that can be targeted. A comprehensive treatment algorithm for HE should include prompt diagnosis and treatment of infections and/or bleeding, optimal electrolyte, acid-base and volume management, nutritional support to improve sarcopenia, replenishment of various vitamins and microelements, and tight glycemic control. Future therapies will likely include modulation of the gut microbiome, reduction of systemic inflammation, and more specific neurotransmitter targets.

DISCLOSURE

The authors have nothing to disclose.

REFERENCES

1. Alsahhar J, Rahimi R. Updates on the pathophysiology and therapeutic targets for hepatic encephalopathy. CurrOpinGastroenterol 2019;35(3):145–54.
2. Fichet J, Mercier E, Genée O, et al. Prognosis and 1-year mortality of intensive care unit patients with severe hepatic encephalopathy. J CritCare 2009;24: 364–70.
3. Bajaj JS, Wade JB, Gibson DP, et al. The multi-dimensional burden of cirrhosis and hepatic encephalopathy on patients and caregivers. Am J Gastroenterol 2011;106(9):1646–53.
4. Vilstrup H, Amodio P, Bajaj J, et al. Hepatic encephalopathy in chronic liver disease: 2014 practice guideline by the American Association for the Study of Liver Diseases and the European Association for the Study of the Liver. Hepatology 2014;60:715.
5. Cordoba J, Lopez-HellinPlanas J, Planas M, et al. Normal protein diet for episodic hepatic encephalopathy: results of a randomized study. J Hepatol 2004;41(1): 38–43.
6. Montano-Loza AJ, Meza-Junco J, Prado CM, et al. Muscle wasting is associated with mortality in patients with cirrhosis. ClinGastroenterolHepatol 2012;10(2): 166–73.
7. Uribe M, Márquez MA, Garcia Ramos G, et al. Treatment of chronic portal–systemic encephalopathy with vegetable and animal protein diets.A controlled crossover study. Dig Dis Sci 1982;27(12):1109–16.
8. Han K-H. Mechanisms of the effects of acidosis and hypokalemia on renal ammonia metabolism. ElectrolyteBlood Press 2011;9(2):45–9.

9. Nagami GT. Enhanced ammonia secretion by proximal tubules from mice receiving NH4Cl: role of angiotensin II. Am J Physiol Renal Physiol 2002; 282(3):F472–7.
10. Jalan R, Kapoor D. Enhanced renal ammonia excretion following volume expansion in patients with well compensated cirrhosis of the liver. Gut 2003;52(7): 1041–5.
11. Dasarathy S, Mookerjee RP, Rackayova V, et al. Ammonia toxicity: from head to toe? MetabBrain Dis 2017;32(2):529–38.
12. Weiner ID, Mitch WE, Sands JM. Urea and ammonia metabolism and the control of renal nitrogen excretion. Clin J Am SocNephrol 2015;10(8):1444–58.
13. Desjardins P, Rao KV, Michalak A, et al. Effect of portacaval anastomosis on glutamine synthetase protein and gene expression in brain, liver and skeletal muscle. MetabBrain Dis 1999;14(4):273–80.
14. Merli M, Giusto M, Lucidi C, et al. Muscle depletion increases the risk of overt and minimal hepatic encephalopathy: results of a prospective study. MetabBrain Dis 2013;28:281–4.
15. Jawaro T, Yang A, Dixit D, et al. Management of hepatic encephalopathy: a primer. Ann Pharmacother 2016;50:569–77.
16. Gluud LL, Dam G, Les I, et al. Branched-chain amino acids for people with hepatic encephalopathy. CochraneDatabaseSyst Rev 2017;(5):CD001939.
17. Kircheis G, Nilius R, Held C, et al. Therapeutic efficacy of L-ornithine-L- aspartate infusions in patients with cirrhosis and hepatic encephalopathy: results of a placebo-controlled, double- blind study. Hepatology 1997;25:1351–60.
18. Rockey DC, Vierling JM, Mantry P, et al. Randomized, double-blind, controlled study of glycerol phenylbutyrate in hepatic encephalopathy HALT-HE Study Group. Hepatology 2014;59(3):1073–83.
19. Ventura-Cots M, Concepción M, Arranz JA. Impact of ornithine phenylacetate (OCR-002) in lowering plasma ammonia after upper gastrointestinal bleeding in cirrhotic patients. TherapAdvGastroenterol 2016;9(6):823–35.
20. Takuma Y, Nouso K, Makino Y, et al. Clinical trial: oral zinc in hepatic encephalopathy. Aliment PharmacolTher 2010;32:1080–90.
21. Chavez-Tapia NC, Cesar-Arce A, Barrientos-Gutierrez T, et al. A systematic review and meta-analysis of the use of oral zinc in the treatment of hepatic encephalopathy. Nutr J 2013;12:74.
22. Kikeri D, Sun A, Zeidel ML, et al. Cell membranes impermeable to NH3. Nature 1989;339:478–80.
23. Bakouh N, Benjelloun F, Cherif-Zahar B, et al. The challenge of understanding ammonium homeostasis and the role of the Rh glycoproteins. TransfusClinBiol 2006;13:139–46.
24. Saparov SM, Liu K, Agre P, et al. Fast and selective ammonia transport by aquaporin-8. J BiolChem 2007;282:5296–301.
25. Felipo V, Butterworth RF. Neurobiology of ammonia. ProgNeurobiol 2002;67(4): 259–79.
26. Poveda MJ, Bernabeu A, Concepción L, et al. Brain edema dynamics in patients with overt hepatic encephalopathy: a magnetic resonance imaging study. Neuroimage 2010;52:481–7.
27. Aggarwal S, Kramer D, Yonas H, et al. Cerebral hemodynamic and metabolic changes in fulminant hepatic failure: a retrospective study. Hepatology 1994; 19(1):80–7.
28. Albrecht J, Norenberg MD. Glutamine: a Trojan horse in ammonia neurotoxicity. Hepatology 2006;44(4):788–94.

29. Umapathy S, Dhiman RK, Grover S, et al. Persistence of cognitive impairment after resolution of overt hepatic encephalopathy. Am J Gastroenterol 2014;109(7):1011–9.
30. Guevara M, Baccaro ME, Torre A, et al. Hyponatremia is a risk factor of hepatic encephalopathy in patients with cirrhosis: a prospective study with time-dependent analysis. Am J Gastroenterol 2009;104(6):382–1389.
31. Butterworth R. Hepatic encephalopathy in cirrhosis: pathology and pathophysiology. Drugs 2019;79(Suppl 1):17–21.
32. Butterworth RF. The liver–brain axis in liver failure:neuroinflammation and encephalopathy. Nat Rev GastroenterolHepatol 2013;10:522–8.
33. Cagnin A, Taylor-Robinson SD, Forton DM, et al. In vivo imaging of cerebral "peripheral benzodiazepine binding sites" in patients with hepatic encephalopathy. Gut 2006;55:547–53.
34. Butterworth R. Neuronal cell death in hepatic encephalopathy. MetabBrain Dis 2007;22(3–4):309–20.
35. Ong JP, Aggarwal A, Krieger D, et al. Correlation between ammonia levels and the severity of hepatic encephalopathy. Am J Med 2003;114:188–93.
36. Tilg H, Wilmer A, Vogel W, et al. Serum levels of cytokines in chronic liver disease. Gastroenterology 1992;103:264–74.
37. Merli M, Lucidi C, Pentassuglio I, et al. Increased risk of cognitive impairment in cirrhotic patients with bacterial infections. J Hepatol 2013;59:243–50.
38. Shawcross DL, Davies NA, Williams R, et al. Systemic inflammatory response exacerbates the neuropsychological effects of induced hyperammonemia in cirrhosis. J Hepatol 2004;40:247–54.
39. Bellot P, Francés R, Such J. Pathological bacterial translocation in cirrhosis: pathophysiology, diagnosis and clinical implications. LiverInt 2013;33(1):31–9.
40. Wiest R, Garcia-Tsao G. Bacterial translocation (BT) in cirrhosis. Hepatology 2005;41:422–33.
41. Chavez-Tapia NC, Tellez-Avila FI, Garcia-Leiva J. Use and overuse of proton pump inhibitors in cirrhotic patients. Med SciMonit 2008;14:CR468–72.
42. Dam G, Vilstrup H, Watson H, et al. Proton pump inhibitors as a risk factor for hepatic encephalopathy and spontaneous bacterial peritonitis in patients with cirrhosis with ascites. Hepatology 2016;64:1265–72.
43. Tsai CF, Chen MH, Wang YP, et al. Proton pump inhibitors increase risk for && hepatic encephalopathy in patients with cirrhosis in a population study. Gastroenterology 2017;152:134–41.
44. Odeh M, Sabo E, Srugo I, et al. Relationship between tumor necrosis factor-α and ammonia in patients with hepatic encephalopathy due to chronic liver failure. Ann Med 2005;37:603–12.
45. Chao CC, Hu S. Tumor necrosis factor-alpha potentiates glutamate neucrotoxicity in human fetal brain cell cultures. DevNeurosci 1994;16:172–9.
46. Duchini A, Govindarajan S, Santucci M, et al. Effects of tumor necrosis factor-alpha and interleukin-6 on fluid-phase permeability and ammonia diffusion in CNS-derived endothelial cells. J Investig Med 1996;44(8):474–82.
47. Brian JE Jr, Faraci FM. Tumor necrosis factor-α-induced dilatation of cerebral arterioles. Stroke 1998;29:509–15.
48. Wong F, Bernardi M, Balk R, et al. Sepsis in cirrhosis: report on the 7th meeting of the international ascites club. Gut 2005;54:718–25.
49. Liu Q, Duan ZP, Ha DK, et al. Synbiotic modulation of gut flora: effect on minimal hepatic encephalopathy in patients with cirrhosis. Hepatology 2004;39:1441–9.

50. Ahluwalia V, Betrapally NS, Hylemon PB. Impaired gut-liver-brain axis in patients with cirrhosis. Sci Rep 2016;6:26800.
51. Bajaj JS, Ridlon JM, Hylemon PB, et al. Linkage of gut microbiome with cognition in hepatic encephalopathy. Am J PhysiolGastrointestLiverPhysiol 2012;302: G168–75.
52. Cao Q, Yu CB, ang SG, et al. Effect of probiotic treatment on cirrhotic patients with minimal hepatic encephalopathy: a meta-analysis. HepatobiliaryPancreat Dis Int 2018;17(1):9–16.
53. Bajaj JS, Salzman NH, Acharya C. Fecal microbial transplant capsules are safe in hepatic encephalopathy: a phase 1, randomized, placebo-controlled trial. Hepatology 2019. https://doi.org/10.1002/hep.30690.
54. Butterworth RF. Glutamate transporters in hyperammonemia. NeurochemInt 2002;41(2–3):81–5.
55. Hamberger A, Lindroth P, Nyström B. Regulation of glutamate biosynthesis and release in vitro by low levels of ammonium ions. Brain Res 1982;237:339–50.
56. Raabe W. Effects of NH4+ on reflexes in cat spinal cord. J Neurophysiol 1990;64: 65–574.
57. Fan P, Lavoie J, Le NLO, et al. Neurochemical and electrophysiological studies on the inhibitory effect of ammonium ions on synaptic transmission in slices of rat hippocampus: evidence for a postsynaptic action. Neuroscience 1990;37: 327–34.
58. Palomero-Gallagher N, Zilles K. Neurotransmitter receptor alterations in hepatic encephalopathy: a review. Arch BiochemBiophys 2013;536(2):109–21.
59. Cascino A, Cangiano C, Fiaccadori F, et al. Plasma and cerebrospinal fluid amino acid patterns in hepatic encephalopathy. Dig Dis Sci 1982;27:828–32.
60. Batshaw ML, Heyes M, Djali S, et al. Tryptophan (Trp), quinolinate (QUIN) and serotonin (5-HT). 1. Alterations in children with hyperammonemia (HA). SocNeurosci 1990;323:1.
61. Jellinger K, Riederer P, Kleinberger G, et al. Brain monoamines in human hepatic encephalopathy. ActaNeuropathol 1978;43:63–8.
62. Erecinska M, Pastuszko A, Wilson DF, et al. Ammonia-induced release of neurotransmitters from rat brain synaptosomes: differences between the effects on amines and amino acids. J Neurochem 1987;49:258–1265.
63. Dantzer R, O'Connor JC, Lawson MA, et al. Inflammation-associated depression: from serotonin to kynurenine. Psychoneuroendocrinology 2011;36:26–436.
64. Jones EA. Ammonia, the GABA neurotransmitter system, and hepatic encephalopathy. MetabBrain Dis 2002;17(4):275–81.
65. Ahboucha S, Gamrani H, Baker G. GABAergicneurosteroids: the "endogenous benzodiazepines" of acute liver failure. NeurochemInt 2012;60(7):707–14.
66. Als-Nielsen B, Gluud LL, Gluud C. Benzodiazepine receptor antagonists for hepatic encephalopathy. Cochrane Database Syst Rev 2004;(2):CD002798.
67. Haussinnger D, Sies H. Hepatic encephalopathy. Arch BiochemBiophys 2013; 536(2):97–204.
68. Ahboucha S, Layrargues GP, Mamer O, et al. Increased brain concentrations of a neuroinhibitory steroid in human hepatic encephalopathy. Ann Neurol 2005;58(1): 169–70.
69. Johansson M, Agusti A, Llansola M, et al. V GR3027 antagonizes GABAA receptor-potentiating neurosteroids and restores spatial learning and motor coordination in rats with chronic hyperammonemia and hepatic encephalopathy. Am J PhysiolGastrointestLiver Physiol 2015;309(5):G400–9.

70. Normandin L, Hazell AS. Manganese neurotoxicity: an update of pathophysiologic mechanisms. MetabBrain Dis 2002;17:375–87.
71. Butterworth RF. Neurotransmitter dysfunction in hepatic encephalopathy: new approaches and new findings. MetabBrain Dis 2001;16(1–2):55–65.
72. Bouabid S, Tinakoua A, Lakhdar-Ghazal N, et al. Manganese neurotoxicity: behavior disorders associated with dysfunctions in the basal ganglia and neurochemical transmission. J Neurochem 2016;136:677–91.
73. Burkhard PR, Delavelle J, Du Pasquier R, et al. Chronic parkinsonism associated with cirrhosis: a distinct subset of acquired hepatocerebral degeneration. Arch Neurol 2003;60(4):521–8.
74. Butt Z, Jadoon NA, Salaria ON, et al. Diabetes mellitus and decompensated cirrhosis: risk of hepatic encephalopathy in different age groups. J Diabetes 2013;5:449–55.
75. Jepsen P, Watson H, Andersen PK, et al. Diabetes as a risk factor for hepatic encephalopathy in cirrhosis patients. J Hepatol 2015;63(5):1133–8.
76. Ampuero J, Ranchal I, del Mar Díaz-Herrero M, et al. Role of diabetes mellitus on hepatic encephalopathy. MetabBrain Dis 2013;28:277–9.
77. Ampuero J, Ranchal I, Nuñez D, et al. Metformin inhibits glutaminase activity and protects against hepatic encephalopathy. PLoS One 2012;7:e49279.
78. Magen I, Avraham Y, Ackerman Z, et al. Cannabidiol ameliorates cognitive and motor impairments in mice with bile duct ligation. J Hepatol 2009;51(3):528–34.
79. Abulseoud OA, Zuccoli ML, Zhang L, et al. The acute effect of cannabis on plasma, liver and brain ammonia dynamics, a translational study. EurNeuropsychopharmacol 2017;27(7):679–90.

Clinical Manifestations of Hepatic Encephalopathy

Peter Dellatore, MD[a,b], Maggie Cheung, MD[a,b], Noah Y. Mahpour, MD[a,b], Augustine Tawadros, MD[a,b], Vinod K. Rustgi, MD, MBA[c,*]

KEYWORDS

- Hepatic encephalopathy • Classification • Grading • Clinical manifestations

KEY POINTS

- The clinical presentations of patients with hepatic encephalopathy include a wide range of symptoms with different levels of severity.
- Hepatic encephalopathy is categorized based on 4 main features: the underlying disease, the severity of manifestations, the time course, and whether precipitating factors are present.
- The severity of hepatic encephalopathy is classically identified using the West Haven Criteria, which include 5 grades ranging from minimal (slightly impaired) to grade IV (comatose).
- Other grading scales have proved advantageous and include the Hepatic Encephalopathy Scoring Algorithm, Clinical Hepatic Encephalopathy Staging Scale, and the Glasgow Coma Scale.

INTRODUCTION

Hepatic encephalopathy (HE) is a syndrome occurring in patients with acute-on-chronic liver disease. In many cases, it is difficult to identify the exact onset because the initial symptoms are subtle; however, it remains a clinical landmark in patients with advanced disease.[1] Although it may initially present as minimal symptoms that can be managed, it is associated with a poor prognosis, because patients that progress to severe HE have increased mortality, with some studies showing an increase of greater than 50% mortality in the first year alone.[2,3] The symptoms of HE mainly affect the patient's mental status, musculoskeletal system, and mood/behavior.[4] These symptoms have a wide spectrum of severity, but can initially be very mild, so much so that most of these patients first present to their primary care physicians or neurologists rather than

[a] Department of Internal Medicine, Rutgers-Robert Wood Johnson Medical School, 125 Paterson Street, New Brunswick, NJ 08901, USA; [b] Department of Medicine, 125 Paterson Street, New Brunswick, NJ 08901, USA; [c] Department Gastroenterology and Hepatology, Rutgers-Robert Wood Johnson Medical School, 125 Paterson Street, Suite 5100B, New Brunswick, NJ 08901, USA
* Corresponding author.
E-mail address: vr262@rwjms.rutgers.edu

Clin Liver Dis 24 (2020) 189–196
https://doi.org/10.1016/j.cld.2020.01.010
1089-3261/20/© 2020 Elsevier Inc. All rights reserved.

liver.theclinics.com

liver specialists.[1] Given the many presentations, multiple grading scales and criteria have been developed to better assess the symptoms and overall clinical status of each individual patient.

CLINICAL MANIFESTATIONS

HE produces a wide spectrum of neurologic, psychiatric, and musculoskeletal symptoms. Many patients with only minimal or early-stage encephalopathy simply report disturbances in their sleep-wake cycles.[5] In patients that are seemingly asymptomatic, suspected deficits may be detected with specialized tests designed to uncover subtle mental status changes.[6] These tests include psychometric testing of attention, working memory, psychomotor speed, and visuospatial ability.[7,8] More specifically, this includes a myriad of neuropsychological or neuropsychometric tests that use either paper-and-pencil or computerized tests.[9] These tests include the Psychometric Hepatic Encephalopathy Score, The Repeatable Battery for the Assessment of Neuropsychological Status, Inhibitory Control Test, Cognitive Drug Research, Scan Test, and the Stroop App Test.[9] Although these tests are promising given their high sensitivity and low cost, they are limited by time, the necessity of trained test administrators, and results that are affected by the patient's age and baseline education.[9]

As the symptoms of HE progress, patients commonly show personality changes, such as apathy, disinhibition, and irritability.[10,11] In many cases, the patients do not report these symptoms themselves, but family members or close friends may bring up their concerns. Ultimately, if not treated, these psychological symptoms turn into cognitive impairments, including, but not limited to, disorientation, memory impairment, slurred speech, confusion, and shortened attention span.[10,11] The recent International Society for Hepatic Encephalopathy and Nitrogen Metabolism (ISHEN) article uses the onset of disorientation or asterixis as the initial mark of overt HE.

Patients also show musculoskeletal symptoms that are secondary to motor system abnormalities. As with neuropsychiatric symptoms, the presentation of neuromuscular symptoms is based on the severity of HE. Patients with minimally affected physical capacities may show altered handwriting or issues with coordination.[12] The hallmark of early to middle stages of HE is asterixis. Asterixis is described as a flapping tremor; however, this is not a true tremor but a negative myoclonus that results in loss of postural tone. It is caused by abnormal function of the diencephalic motor centers that regulate the tone of paired agonist/antagonist muscles.[13] It is most commonly elicited when patients hyperextend their wrists, but it can be observed in the patient's feet, legs, arms, tongue, and eyelids.[12] Although it is the physical examination finding most attributed to HE, it is not pathognomonic, because it can be seen in other clinical entities, such as uremia.[14] In its most severe form, HE-induced musculoskeletal changes can lead to hyperreflexia, clonus, and rigidity.[12] In cases of persistent HE, cirrhosis-related parkinsonism symptoms may occur, resulting in extrapyramidal symptoms, including masked facies, rigidity, bradykinesia, slowed speech, and parkinsonian tremors.[14,15] Unlike other manifestations of HE, the parkinsonism symptoms have a distinct feature in that they are irreversible.[12] However, these permanent symptoms are more prevalent than was previously thought and are seen in approximately 4% of cases.[15]

CLASSIFICATION

It is difficult to assess the clinical status of each patient given the many symptoms and vast range of severity of presentations. To further complicate the matter, neuromuscular symptoms do not parallel those of neuropsychiatric or cognitive symptoms. In an attempt to better classify HE, multiple grading scales and classification schemes have been developed.

HE is categorized based on 4 features: the underlying disease, the severity of manifestations, the time course, and whether precipitating factors are present.[16,17] The first classification criterion is based on the underlying cause of HE. Type A is HE in the setting of acute liver failure, type B is in the setting of portal-systemic bypass with no intrinsic hepatocellular disease, and type C is in the setting of cirrhosis with portal hypertension or systemic shunting.[16,17] The most commonly occurring type is type C,[18] and although not truly a sign of HE, patients who have type C HE frequently also show clinical signs of liver failure, such as jaundice, ascites, spider telangiectasias, and palmar erythema, among other manifestations.[19]

With regard to severity, patients can be graded by using the West Haven Criteria (WHC), which range from minimal to grade IV (**Table 1**). In minimal HE (MHE), there are simply abnormal results on psychometric or neurophysiologic testing without clinical manifestations. In grade I, patients show changes in their behavior, with mild confusion, slurred speech, and disturbances in their sleep-wake cycles. Grade II is defined by lethargy and worsening confusion. Grade III is dramatic worsening of grade II, with stupor, incoherent speech, and somnolence. In addition, the patients should be considered for grade IV when they are in a nonresponsive state, or coma.[12,16,17]

The defining physical examination feature of MHE is impaired handwriting, whereas grade I shows uncoordinated initiation of motor movements. Grade II is signified by asterixis. Notably, the signs of asterixis weaken in grade III, and disappear in grade IV, because patients at those grades can show decerebrate or decorticate posturing, masking signs of asterixis.[20] Grade IV is defined by hyporeflexia and ataxia, which may eventually degrade to hyperreflexia, clonus, and rigidity. The final and most severe physical examination findings of HE are opisthotonus and coma.[12,20]

Table 1
West Haven criteria

Grade	Clinical Features
Grade 0	• Unimpaired
Grade 1	• Trivial lack of awareness • Shortened attention span • Impairment of addition or subtraction • Euphoria or anxiety • Altered sleep rhythm
Grade II	• Lethargy or apathy • Inappropriate behavior • Disorientation for time • Personality change • Asterixis • Dyspraxia
Grade III	• Somnolence to semistupor • Confused • Gross disorientation • Bizarre behavior
Grade IV	• Coma

From American Association for the Study of Liver, D. and L. European Association for the Study of the, Hepatic encephalopathy in chronic liver disease: 2014 practice guideline by the European Association for the Study of the Liver and the American Association for the Study of Liver Diseases. J Hepatol, 2014. **61**(3): p. 642-59; with permission.

Patients are further classified according to time course and whether it was precipitated or not.[12] Timing is further broken down into categories of episodic, recurrent, or persistent. To classify as recurrent, bouts of HE must occur within intervals of less than 6 months, whereas persistent entails altered behavior that is always present in the setting of recurrent HE.[12]

The final classification revolves around precipitating factors for the episode of HE. In type C, nearly all cases have an identifiable precipitating factor that is essential to determine for treatment.[12] Examples of precipitating factors include infections, gastrointestinal bleeding, overdiuresis, electrolyte abnormalities, and constipation.[12]

GRADING

As detailed earlier, the WHC were among the first efforts to better categorize the severity of HE, ranging grade 0 to grade IV, as detailed in **Table 1**. However, a criticism of the WHC is that there is significant interobserver and intraobserver variability when in use, given that it relies on the physician's interpretation of patient symptoms and the ability to detect subtle changes in patient behavior. This variability results in subjectivity, lack of specific definitions for assessing dysfunctions, and an imprecise ability to differentiate between early and late HE.[21] The Hepatic Encephalopathy Scoring Algorithm (HESA) was developed to provide a more reliable grading of severity of HE by combining both subjective and objective data.[21] It accomplished this by minimizing the effects of age and education on patients' overall scores and testing.[22] The HESA has 4 grades of severity of HE, with 1 being the least severe and 4 being the most severe. The scale divides symptoms to be assessed by clinical judgment and by neuropsychological testing (**Table 2**). Based on the grade of HE, it relies more on either clinical examination or neuropsychological testing. For example, in higher grades in which neuropsychological testing is not appropriate, the HESA relies more on the clinical examination.[22] If the patient fulfills a certain number of clinical indicators, the patient is categorized into the appropriate grade. For grade 4, patients must have all 3 clinical indicators: no opening of eyes, reaction to simple commands, and no verbal or voice response. Patients are considered to have grade 3 HE if they have 3 or more of the following: somnolence, confusion, disorientation to place, bizarre behavior, and motor abnormalities. Patients are considered grade 2 if they have 2 or more of the clinical indicators of lethargy, inappropriate behavior, disorientation to time, slurred speech, and hyperactive reflexes, and 3 or more of the neuropsychological indicators of anxiety, slow response, amnesia, and impaired simple addition and subtraction. Patients are considered grade 1 if they have 4 or more of the following: sleep impairment, tremor, impaired complex computations, shortened attention span, impaired construction ability, euphoria, and depression.[21]

Multiples studies have shown promising data with regard to HESA. In a study to determine the efficacy of rifaximin for the maintenance of remission, HESA had good precision in differentiating grades 0, 1, and 2.[23] In another study identifying HE grading scales across many sites, there was no significant variability, showing the strong inter-rater reliability of HESA.[24] Ultimately, more data are needed to validate HESA, but, with the combination of both clinical indicators and objective neuropsychological indicators, it can provide a more sensitive grading system for HE, particularly in patients with mild HE.

Another scale constructed to assess the severity of HE is the Clinical Hepatic Encephalopathy Staging Scale (CHESS). CHESS consists of 9 clinical items, and determines severity in a linear fashion rather than using specific grades like the WHC and the HESA.[24] The scale is more intuitive, using simple terms and questions, and

Table 2
Hepatic Encephalopathy Scoring Algorithm

Grade 4	○ No eyes opening □ No reaction to simple commands If all applicable → grade 4 HE	○ No verbal or voice response to stimulation If not, proceed below	
Grade 3	○ Somnolence ○ Bizarre behavior/anger □ Mental control = ○ using the Wechsler Memory Scale If 3 or more applicable → grade 3 HE	○ Confusion ○ Motor abnormalities: clonus, rigidity, nystagmus, Babinski If not, proceed below	○ Disorientation to place
Grade 2	○ Lethargy ○ Hyperactive reflexes □ Slow responses □ Anxiety If 2 or more ○ and 3 or more □ → grade 2	○ Loss of time ○ Inappropriate behavior □ Amnesia of recent events □ Impaired simple computations If not, proceed below	○ Slurred speech
Grade 1	○ Impaired sleep/wake cycle □ Impaired complex computations Impaired construction ability If 4 or more applicable → grade I	○ Tremor □ Shortened attention span □ Euphoria or depression If not, patient is grade 0	

○, Symptom determined by clinical judgment; □, symptom determined by neuropsychological test
Data from Hassanein, T.I., R.C. Hilsabeck, and W. Perry, *Introduction to the Hepatic Encephalopathy Scoring Algorithm (HESA).* Dig Dis Sci, 2008. **53**(2): p. 529-38.

Table 3
Clinical Hepatic Encephalopathy Staging Scale

		1 Point	0 Points
1	Does the patient know which month it is?	Yes	No or cannot talk
2	Does the patient know which day of the week it is?	Yes	No or cannot talk
3	Can the patient count backward from 10 to 1 without making mistakes or stopping?	Yes	No or cannot talk
4	If asked to do so, can the patient raise their arms	Yes	No or cannot talk
5	Does the patient understand what you are saying?	Yes	No or cannot talk
6	Is the patient awake and alert?	Yes	No or cannot talk
7	Is the patient fast asleep and it is difficult to arouse them?	Yes	No or cannot talk
8	Can the patient talk?	Yes	No or cannot talk
9	Can the patient talk correctly? Are you able to understand them?	Yes	No or cannot talk

From Sakamoto, M., et al., Assessment and usefulness of clinical scales for semiquantification of overt hepatic encephalopathy. Clin Liver Dis, 2012. **16**(1): p. 27-42; with permission.

Table 4
Glasgow Coma Scale by hepatic encephalopathy grade as determined by Hepatic Encephalopathy Scoring Algorithm

Grade of HE	Median GCS Score (Range)
IV	3 (3–12)
III	11 (3–15)
II	14 (3–15)
I	15 (11–15)
Minimal	15 (11–15)

From Sakamoto, M., et al., Assessment and usefulness of clinical scales for semiquantification of overt hepatic encephalopathy. Clin Liver Dis, 2012. 16(1): p. 27-42; with permission.

dichotomic answers (**Table 3**). Patients are given a point if they do not satisfy the specific item, and the total points indicate the severity of HE, with 0 being unimpaired and 9 being in a coma.[24] The simple wording also allows for translation into different languages, helping facilitate assessment of HE in patients who do not speak English.[24] Although CHESS has been shown to have internal consistency and reproducibility, it is not widely used and still needs to be validated with other centers.[25]

Glasgow Coma Scale (GCS) is another tool that can be used in HE. Aside from being the universal standard for assessing mental status in patients with traumatic brain injury, it is helpful in cases of severe HE, specifically grades III and IV.[22] The GCS has been found to correlate with both the HESA and CHESS.[21,24] Although there is correlation between the HE grades and GCS, as shown in **Table 4**, multiple GCS scores overlap with each grade, particularly with lower-grade HE. Hence GCS is solely used except in patients with severe HE.

SUMMARY

The clinical presentation of HE includes a wide range of symptoms with different levels of severity. These symptoms mainly affect the neurologic, psychiatric, and musculoskeletal systems. Symptoms may be as subtle as disturbances in the sleep-wake cycle,[5] or may be as severe as a coma.[12,16,17] The primary personality changes include apathy, disinhibition, and irritability; cognitive impairments include, but are not limited to, disorientation, memory impairment, slurred speech, confusion, and shortened attention span.[10,11] Musculoskeletal symptoms also vary dramatically based on the severity of HE the patient is experiencing. Patients with minimally affected physical capacities may show altered handwriting or issues with coordination, whereas patients who become more impaired show asterixis, hyporeflexia, and ataxia. In its most severe form, HE-induced musculoskeletal changes can lead to hyperreflexia, clonus, and rigidity.[12]

Because of the various presentations, classification schemes are used to better categorize patients with HE. It is categorized based on 4 main features: the underlying disease, the severity of manifestations, the time course, and whether precipitating factors are present.[16,17] The severity of the manifestations is classically identified using the WHC, which include 5 grades ranging from MHE to grade IV. Patients with MHE are grossly unimpaired. Grade I presents as incoordination, grade II as asterixis, grade III with stupor, and grade IV presents as coma.[12,21,22,24] Although WHC is the mainstay, several other grading scales exist. These scales include HESA, CHESS, and the GCS. Each has its own advantages. For example, the HESA is arguably more objective than the WHC and results in strong inter-rater reliability to provide a more sensitive grading system for HE, particularly mild HE.[21,22,24] CHESS is a simple test that has been shown to have internal consistency and reproducibility.[24] Although not originally intended for HE, GCS can be used to help further classify patients with severe HE. Each provides additional data in the assessment of patients, but they require more validation before universal clinical implementation.

DISCLOSURE

The authors have nothing to disclose.

REFERENCES

1. Wijdicks EF. Hepatic encephalopathy. N Engl J Med 2016;375(17):1660–70.
2. Fichet J, et al. Prognosis and 1-year mortality of intensive care unit patients with severe hepatic encephalopathy. J Crit Care 2009;24(3):364–70.
3. Garcia-Martinez R, Simon-Talero M, Cordoba J. Prognostic assessment in patients with hepatic encephalopathy. Dis Markers 2011;31(3):171–9.
4. Mas A. Hepatic encephalopathy: from pathophysiology to treatment. Digestion 2006;73(Suppl 1):86–93.
5. Cordoba J, et al. High prevalence of sleep disturbance in cirrhosis. Hepatology 1998;27(2):339–45.
6. Khungar V, Poordad F. Hepatic encephalopathy. Clin Liver Dis 2012;16(2): 301–20.
7. Amodio P, et al. Characteristics of minimal hepatic encephalopathy. Metab Brain Dis 2004;19(3–4):253–67.
8. McCrea M, et al. Neuropsychological characterization and detection of subclinical hepatic encephalopathy. Arch Neurol 1996;53(8):758–63.
9. Nabi E, Bajaj JS. Useful tests for hepatic encephalopathy in clinical practice. Curr Gastroenterol Rep 2014;16(1):362.
10. Weissenborn K. Diagnosis of encephalopathy. Digestion 1998;59(Suppl 2):22–4.
11. Wiltfang J, et al. Psychiatric aspects of portal-systemic encephalopathy. Metab Brain Dis 1998;13(4):379–89.
12. American Association for the Study of Liver Diseases, European Association for the Study of the Liver. Hepatic encephalopathy in chronic liver disease: 2014 practice guideline by the European Association for the study of the liver and the American Association for the Study of liver diseases. J Hepatol 2014;61(3): 642–59.
13. Timmermann L, et al. Mini-asterixis in hepatic encephalopathy induced by pathologic thalamo-motor-cortical coupling. Neurology 2003;61(5):689–92.
14. Weissenborn K, et al. Neurological and neuropsychiatric syndromes associated with liver disease. AIDS 2005;19(Suppl 3):S93–8.
15. Tryc AB, et al. Cirrhosis-related Parkinsonism: prevalence, mechanisms and response to treatments. J Hepatol 2013;58(4):698–705.
16. Ferenci P, et al. Hepatic encephalopathy–definition, nomenclature, diagnosis, and quantification: final report of the working party at the 11th World Congresses of Gastroenterology, Vienna, 1998. Hepatology 2002;35(3):716–21.
17. Frederick RT. Current concepts in the pathophysiology and management of hepatic encephalopathy. Gastroenterol Hepatol (N Y) 2011;7(4):222–33.
18. Bajaj JS, Wade JB, Sanyal AJ. Spectrum of neurocognitive impairment in cirrhosis: Implications for the assessment of hepatic encephalopathy. Hepatology 2009;50(6):2014–21.

19. Mumtaz K, et al. Precipitating factors and the outcome of hepatic encephalopathy in liver cirrhosis. J Coll Physicians Surg Pak 2010;20(8):514–8.
20. Basu PP, Shah NJ. Clinical and neurologic manifestation of minimal hepatic encephalopathy and overt hepatic encephalopathy. Clin Liver Dis 2015;19(3): 461–72.
21. Hassanein TI, Hilsabeck RC, Perry W. Introduction to the hepatic encephalopathy scoring algorithm (HESA). Dig Dis Sci 2008;53(2):529–38.
22. Sakamoto M, et al. Assessment and usefulness of clinical scales for semiquantification of overt hepatic encephalopathy. Clin Liver Dis 2012;16(1):27–42.
23. Shayto RH, Abou Mrad R, Sharara AI. Use of rifaximin in gastrointestinal and liver diseases. World J Gastroenterol 2016;22(29):6638–51.
24. Ortiz M, et al. Development of a clinical hepatic encephalopathy staging scale. Aliment Pharmacol Ther 2007;26(6):859–67.
25. Cordoba J. New assessment of hepatic encephalopathy. J Hepatol 2011;54(5): 1030–40.

Laboratory Abnormalities of Hepatic Encephalopathy

Briette Verken Karanfilian, MD[a,b], Maggie Cheung, MD[a,b], Peter Dellatore, MD[a,b], Taeyang Park, MD[a,b], Vinod K. Rustgi, MD, MBA[c,*]

KEYWORDS

- Hepatic encephalopathy • Diagnostic testing • Imaging • Ammonia
- Magnetic resonance spectroscopy • Electroencephalogram

KEY POINTS

- Hepatic encephalopathy (HE) is a clinical diagnosis that is obtained through the history and physical examination.
- There is not a serologic test or imaging modality to accurately diagnose HE and assess its severity.
- Ammonia is commonly used, but is not specific to HE, does not correlate with severity, and is easily influenced by testing methods.
- Although there are imaging modalities that offer some insight into cases of HE, they are largely noncontributory and not recommended for diagnosis or assessing severity.

INTRODUCTION

Currently, no gold standard diagnostic laboratory test exists for hepatic encephalopathy (HE).[1] Making the diagnosis of HE involves conducting a thorough history and physical examination to detect the cognitive and neuropsychiatric impairments that define the disease, as well as evaluating for precipitating factors that could have led to its onset.[2] The newer HE grading system put forth by the International Society for Hepatic Encephalopathy and Nitrogen Metabolism was designed with the intent to better standardize the way in which HE is diagnosed. In theory, further standardization of this diagnostic process could involve the use of laboratory studies, including bloodwork and imaging.

In 2014, the American Association for the Study of Liver Diseases (AASLD) and the European Association for the Study of the Liver (EASL) released joint practice guidelines for HE, including information on diagnostic testing. Although several laboratory

[a] Department of Internal Medicine, Rutgers-Robert Wood Johnson Medical School, New Brunswick, NJ, USA; [b] Department of Medicine, 125 Paterson Street, New Brunswick, NJ 08901, USA; [c] Department Gastroenterology and Hepatology, Rutgers-Robert Wood Johnson Medical School, 125 Paterson Street, Suite 5100B, New Brunswick, NJ 08901, USA
* Corresponding author.
E-mail address: vr262@rwjms.rutgers.edu

Clin Liver Dis 24 (2020) 197–208
https://doi.org/10.1016/j.cld.2020.01.011
1089-3261/20/© 2020 Elsevier Inc. All rights reserved.

liver.theclinics.com

and imaging testing modalities exist, and when combined can assist with diagnosis of HE, they have limited diagnostic utility as separate entities and limited utility outside the context of patients' clinical presentations.[1]

SERUM TESTING

Patients can present with HE in the setting of acute liver failure or cirrhosis, and depending on the clinical scenario, they will have laboratory abnormalities commonly associated with liver disease. For instance, cirrhotic patients will have thrombocytopenia, hypoalbuminemia, and elevated international normalized ratio (INR), reflecting decreased synthetic function of the liver. These patients may also have electrolyte disturbances, such as hyponatremia and hypokalemia, and of course, will likely also have a moderate transaminitis. The Model for End-stage Liver Disease (MELD) score, which requires INR, serum bilirubin, and creatinine, is commonly followed in patients with HE, as these patients have significant liver disease and the MELD provides an estimation of disease severity.[3] When considering bloodwork for patients being evaluated for HE, it is critical to rule out other metabolic or toxic causes of encephalopathy, such as electrolyte disturbances, hypercarbia, hypoxemia, sepsis, and medication side effects.[1]

One of the blood tests classically associated with HE itself is an elevated ammonia level (an arterial, venous, or plasma sample). Ammonia is produced in the gastrointestinal tract and released into the portal vein, at which point a normally functioning liver clears most of the ammonia from the bloodstream. However, in those with liver disease, this clearing is impaired, and the ammonia ends up in the systemic circulation. Although there are other toxin imbalances in HE, such as cerebral manganese deposition, this high level of circulating ammonia is the neurotoxin that is thought to precipitate the disease process.[4] It is well known that ammonia should not be used to screen for HE in asymptomatic patients; however, measuring ammonia levels in the diagnostic workup for symptomatic patients remains somewhat controversial. One of the reasons that measurement of ammonia is controversial, and oftentimes considered unreliable, is that there are multiple other reasons why patients may have elevated ammonia levels. For example, ammonia levels can be elevated as a result of urinary tract infections of urease-producing organisms, gastrointestinal bleeding, shock, renal disease, portosystemic shunting, parenteral nutrition, salicylate intoxication, medications, and alcohol.[2] Another reason that ammonia levels are not considered to be an ideal testing modality is that blood ammonia levels do not correlate well with the grading severity of the HE.[5] In addition, the manner in which ammonia samples are collected and handled can influence test results. For instance, the amount of time before the sample is placed on ice or the use of a tourniquet or fist clenching can during blood collection can affect results.[2]

Overall, the practice guidelines put forth by the AASLD and the EASL in 2014 state that increased blood ammonia level alone does not help with diagnosis or prognosis of HE. It is the elevated ammonia in combination with the clinical picture of HE that can be informative.[6] Data have shown that in this context, either venous or arterial ammonia samples can be used with equal accuracy in detecting elevated level.[5] The guidelines also state that because an elevated ammonia level is relatively sensitive in detecting HE, if a patient with purported HE has a normal ammonia level, the accuracy of the diagnosis should be questioned.[1] In addition, if a patient is being treated with an ammonia-lowering drug, repeated measurements of the ammonia level can be helpful in gauging if the treatment is working, although again, the levels do not necessarily correlate with the grading of the HE.[1]

Recently, one other serum marker was proposed: 3-nitrotyrosine. This molecule is a derivative of nitric oxide, which has been implicated as one of the toxins involved in the development of HE.[7] A study by Montoliu and colleagues[7] in 2011 showed that 3-nitro-tyrosine is elevated in patients with minimal HE (MHE). By using a cutoff of 14 nM, they demonstrated that 3-nitrotyrosine was 93% sensitive and 89% specific for diagnosing MHE. At this time, there is still a lack of further research regarding the reliability of this potential marker both for patients with MHE and for patients with overt HE.

IMAGING
Computed Tomography in Hepatic Encephalopathy

In addition to blood testing, patients who present with altered mental status (AMS) in the setting of cirrhosis are likely to undergo head computed tomography (CT) before and during hospital admission.[8] Although CT findings are largely unremarkable, there are subtle findings that suggest frontal cortical atrophy and mild cerebral edema.[9] In a retrospective cohort study, Rahimi and Rockey[10] was found that head CTs in patients with HE have no effect on clinical outcome. Of 1218 patients with cirrhosis with AMS who presented to the emergency room over 3 years, 349 had AMS, with HE being the most common cause (164 of 349).[10] Unless there was a focal neurologic deficit on physical examination, there were no focal findings on any of the head CTs, but rather nonspecific findings or atrophy.[10] These findings were further confirmed by Kumar and colleagues,[11] who found that 67 patients with HE over 3 years had negative head CTs unless there were focal deficits attributed to other etiologies. Furthermore, head CT did not have a correlation with serum studies, such as ammonia, sodium, creatinine, bilirubin, albumin, platelet count, INR, encephalopathy grade, or MELD score.[11] Neither study found a difference in clinical outcome in those who received head CT compared with those who did not, indicating that it may be an unnecessary test unless focal deficits are present.[10,11]

Although head CT may not affect clinical outcome, it is being investigated in critically ill patients as a marker of brain volume. Liotta and colleagues[12] found that changes in intracranial cerebrospinal fluid volume between sequential CT scans could be used as a biomarker of acute brain volume change. Using this, it was discovered that acute declines in osmolality were associated with brain swelling and neurologic deterioration in those with HE. In an attempt to reduce cerebral edema, 11 patients in the intensive care unit being treated for severe cerebral edema in the setting of acute on chronic liver disease received 23.4% hypertonic saline.[13] It was found to increase total cerebrospinal fluid, ventricular volumes, and Glasgow Coma Scale Scores, consistent with a reduction in brain tissue volume.[13]

CT imaging does not demonstrate any focal abnormalities to aid in the diagnosis or clinical outcome in patients with HE.[8,10,11] However, their use to evaluate cerebrospinal fluid and ventricular volumes may provide utility in assessing cerebral edema in severe HE.[12,13]

Positron Emission Computed Tomography

PET is not widely used because of cost, and it is not always available; however, it does provide valuable insight into the pathogenesis of HE. PET can be used to calculate blood flow, glucose metabolism, and ammonia metabolism while specifically identifying cerebral ammonia metabolism and glucose utilization.[14–16] Using PET, it has been discovered that HE results in decreased oxygen consumption and cerebral blood flow in all cortical areas.[17,18] This results in poor neuropsychiatric test performance as seen clinically in HE. More specifically, there was impaired perfusion in the superior prefrontal cortex and increased perfusion in the thalamus, brainstem, medial temporal cortex, and the hippocampus when compared with healthy controls.[19] Another study found significant hypoperfusion in the superior and middle frontal gyri, and inferior parietal lobules compared with the control group.[20]

From a prognostic standpoint, it was found that cerebral perfusion in the superior prefrontal cortex correlated negatively with MELD score.[19] Therefore, PET scans may not be widely available, cost-efficient, or necessary in the diagnostic workup of patients with HE, but they do provide interesting information regarding the pathophysiology of HE that may result in altered neuropsychiatric examinations.

MRI

MRI is a noninvasive tool that can provide valuable information about cell structure, water content, and metabolism in HE. However, it is not routinely used in clinical practice, as there is no consensus in its use in diagnosis of HE with MRI.

T1-weighted MRI

One common finding on T1-weighted (T1W) MRI of patients with HE is bilateral and symmetric hyperintensity of the globus pallidus. Many studies have shown correlation between T1W signal hyperintensity and blood manganese level.[21,22] Manganese accumulation in the brain can be detected as an areas of high signal intensity on T1W images due to T1 shortening by the paramagnetic effects of manganese ion, particularly in the globus pallidus in a bilateral and symmetric fashion.[23] One study demonstrated that contrast measurements in the globus pallidus were greater in patients with neuropsychiatric dysfunction than in those who were unimpaired, and these measurements also correlated with blood ammonia levels.[24] In Krieger and colleagues,[25] compared with those who received elective sclerotherapy, patients who had received transjugular intrahepatic portosystemic shunt had increased hyperresonant globus pallidus on MRI and also exhibited advancing HE. One explanation for this phenomenon is that excess manganese is removed via the hepatobiliary system, and thus in severe disease, it becomes accumulated in the body. Its accumulation in the brain not only causes toxic effects on the dopaminergic neurotransmitter system, but it has been suggested that it can cause deleterious effects on the glutamatergic neurotransmitter system by working synergistically with ammonia.[26]

Despite many studies showing a strong correlation between HE and globus pallidus hyperintensity on T1W MRI, others have suggested otherwise. One study showed that abnormally high intensity in the globus pallidus was seen even in patients without cirrhosis and there was no statistically significant correlation between severity of liver disease to the degree of MRI abnormality, but there was a marked improvement in MR appearances seen after successful liver transplantation.[27] One study could not find a statistically significant correlation between globus pallidus signals in T1W images with chronic HE.[28] Another study demonstrated that basal ganglia hyperintensity represents shunt-induced alterations including portal vein thrombosis and cavernous transformation without signs of liver disease, rather than altered liver function or HE.[29] Fukuzawa and colleagues[30] showed that pallidal hyperintensity on MRI was more prominent in patients with idiopathic portal hypertension than in those with liver cirrhosis, and there was no correlation between hyperintensity and severity of liver dysfunction or HE; there was a stronger correlation with portosystemic shunt in portal hypertension than liver cirrhosis. Therefore, although it may be a helpful tool, T1-weighted MRI is not a reliable technique to diagnose HE.

T2-weighted MRI: fluid-attenuated inversion recovery

Fluid-attenuated inversion recovery (FLAIR) is an MRI technique used to suppress cerebrospinal fluid effect on imaging and accentuate periventricular lesions. In patients with HE, fast FLAIR T2-weighted images showed signal intensity along white matter in or around the corticospinal tract very similar to what is seen in amyotrophic lateral sclerosis.[31] This finding may be because patients with HE develop mild brain edema.[32] After liver transplantation, patients not only exhibited improvement in HE, but T2 hyperintensity along the corticospinal tract improved, as well.[31] This further supports the idea that brain edema causes hyperintensity in the corticospinal tract in patients with HE. However, it is important to note that approximately half of healthy adults also had widespread white matter alteration on fast FLAIR, indicating this may be a normal finding.[33] In addition to these changes, focal T2-weighted white matter lesions (WMLs), which resemble lesions seen in different types of cardiovascular small vessel diseases, have been associated with HE. One study showed presence of WML was associated with older age, but not with vascular risk factors, severity of liver function, or psychometric tests.[34] However, a significant reduction of these lesions was seen after liver transplantation.[35] This finding indicates that these lesions are likely reversible damage compatible with brain edema.

T2-weighted MRI: diffusion-weighted imaging

Diffusion-weighted imaging (DWI) is widely used in neuroimaging, especially in detecting acute strokes. DWI detects random movement of water molecules, which is quantified as apparent diffusion coefficient (ADC). This value may be used to quantify low-grade HE and can even be used as a prognostic tool to predict overt HE.[36] Another useful tool is the diffusion tensor imaging that has been used to measure mean diffusivity (MD) and spherical isotropy (CS) to show intracellular and extracellular edema. Using these imaging techniques, various studies have shown that brain edema plays an important role in HE, but there may be discrepancies in the compartment where the edema exists, depending on the acuity of the encephalopathy.

One study showed that patients with chronic liver failure with or without HE had significantly increased mean ADC values in several parts of the brain, suggesting that in chronic liver failure, vasogenic edema may play a role in the pathogenesis of HE.[37] Kale and colleagues[38] demonstrated that in minimal or early HE, there is an increased MD that improved with lactulose therapy, indicating interstitial edema contributing to the encephalopathy. In another study, it was shown that significantly reduced ADC in patients with fulminant hepatic failure indicated cytotoxic nature of the edema.[39] Rai and colleagues[40] showed decreased MD and increased CS in acute liver failure, demonstrating that there was both increased intracellular and extracellular fluid in acute liver failure.

These findings indicate the complex nature in pathogenesis of HE. One explanation for these findings is that the cytotoxic nature of HE is closely linked to ammonia in patients with liver disease.[41] Glutamine synthetase in the astrocytes converts the ammonia into glutamine, which acts as an osmolyte to cause influx of fluids into cells and causes swelling and eventually cell dysfunction that manifests as HE.[42]

Magnetization transfer

Magnetization transfer (MT) is a type of MRI technique in which imaging is created due to contrast between free protons in water molecules and protons bound to macromolecules. It quantifies MT ratio (MTR), which can provide information regarding macromolecular structure in the brain with its interaction with tissue water. Low MTR can reflect myelin and neuronal membrane damage and change in water content.[43]

Multiple studies have demonstrated that patients with cirrhosis had lower MTR than healthy controls.[44,45] Not only that, some studies have shown that there is a correlation between decrease in MTR and worsening degree of HE.[46,47] Goel and colleagues[48] concluded that patients with HE had increased ammonia level and low MTR. One study even induced hyperammonemia in patients with cirrhosis by giving oral amino acid solution and showed that compared with those who received placebo, these patients had worsening changes in neuropsychiatric function, increase in brain glutamine levels, and reduction in MTR.[49] Lactulose and rifaximin treatment, which is widely used to lower blood ammonia levels in patients with HE, was shown to increase MTR,[50] and patients with cirrhosis who received transplantation showed normalization in MTR..[44] These findings once again indicate that brain edema is a key feature in HE, and ammonia and glutamine play a central role in this process.

Functional MRI

Functional MRI (fMRI) is a technique based on assessment of local blood flow and oxygenation changes due to metabolic changes from brain activity. Task-based fMRI is used to identify brain regions that are involved while performing a specific task, whereas resting-state fMRI is used to associate different brain regions that interact at rest. In 2004, Zafiris and colleagues[51] demonstrated that there was an abnormal connection between the inferior parietal cortex and other parts of the brain in patients with HE by using task-based fMRI on these patients while performing critical flicker frequency. In another study, cirrhotic patients were instructed to perform word-reading and color-naming tasks. The results of the fMRI on these patients suggested that the aberrant network of anterior cingulate cortex–prefrontal cortex–parietal lobe–temporal fusiform gyrus may be involved in manifestation of encephalopathy in these patients.[52] Using resting-state fMRI, one study showed right precuneus and left medial prefrontal cortex may explain the cognitive impairment in patients with minimal HE.[53] In 2016, Chen and colleagues[54] compared resting-state fMRI of cirrhotic patients with and without minimal HE and concluded that there may be alterations in coupling between salience network and default mode and central executive networks. fMRI proves to be an important tool in investigating deranged connections in various brain regions in patients with HE.

Magnetic Resonance Spectroscopy

Magnetic resonance spectroscopy (MRS) is an adjunct to MRI that provides information about the biochemical composition of the imaged tissue.[55] It works by identifying various nuclei, most commonly proton (^1H) and 31-phosphorus (^{31}P), to quantify certain metabolites, such as choline, creatine, N-acetyl aspartate, and other amino acids and osmolytes.[56] Ultimately, this allows identification of a compound that is present in a mixture of metabolites and its concentration.[57] Using MRS, it was discovered that there is an increase in glutamine and glutamate peak according to the severity of HE, with a decrease after clinical resolution.[57] In addition, it was found that there is a reduction in intracellular choline and myo-inositol with a correlation to psychometric performance.[58] The increased glutamine is likely secondary to the increased ammonia load that reaches the blood brain barrier and is incorporated to glutamine in the astrocytes.[59] Overall, there are many studies that demonstrate utility in measuring specific metabolites that may be useful in clinically difficult cases; however, normal ranges and diagnostic thresholds are not yet agreed on.[56]

Electroencephalogram

Electroencephalogram (EEG) is an electrophysiological test that monitors electrical activity in the brain and is able to detect abnormalities that may arise in the setting of toxic and metabolic factors.[60] This technique is one of the neurophysiological tests used to facilitate the diagnosis of HE and has been in use since the 1950s.[61] According to the ASLD/EASL practice guidelines, EEG can be used in conjunction with the Portal Systemic Hepatic Encephalopathy Score (PHES) test to diagnose minimal HE (MHE).[1]

Two main components of the EEG are analyzed: rhythmic background activity, which consists of alpha, beta, theta, and delta waves, and transients, which consist of triphasic waves and bursts of intermittent rhythmic delta activity (IRDA). In the early stages of HE, the low-frequency alpha rhythm (8.5 Hz) is disturbed by random theta waves (4–8 Hz). As the severity increases, there is a shift to primarily theta activity with rare occurrence of delta range activity (<4 Hz) and emergence of triphasic waves and bursts of IRDA. With worsening disease, the EEG becomes severely disorganized with theta, delta, and triphasic waves. As patients progress from moderate/severe HE to coma, the EEG is replaced by high-voltage delta activity and eventually a flat EEG.[60,62] In a study by Amodio and colleagues,[63] EEG alterations could predict the occurrence of overt HE (OHE) and mortality.

Another aspect of EEG that is used to assess HE is the mean dominant frequency (MDF), which is the measure of the overall background frequency of the EEG. The MDF is obtained from spectral analysis, a computerized analysis of the digital EEG. Before spectral analysis, interpretation of an EEG relied on visual inspection of the EEG. With development of spectral analysis, not only did it allow for quantification of various EEG components, but it also reduced inter-intra operator-dependent variability that would be seen in visual inspection of the EEG.[64] As patients progress from MHE to OHE, there is significant slowing of the MDF.[60] The MDF has also been found to have prognostic value in determining 12-month and 18-month mortality, both independently and in addition to the MELD score.[65]

In addition to the general changes of rhythmic background activity and decrease in MDF with progression of HE, Olesen and colleagues[66] also looked at variability of EEG in patients with cirrhosis using continuous wavelet transform and sample entropy. Results showed increased variability in patients with minimal HE, and then eventual loss of variability in patients with OHE.

Sensitivity and specificity of EEG depends on both modality of data analysis and the severity of HE. In the use of visual EEG for diagnosing OHE, sensitivity has been reported to be 57% to 100%, and specificity 41% to 88%.[67–69] With spectral analysis, sensitivity and specificity for overt HE have been reported to be 43% to 100% and 65% to 91%, respectively.[68,70] Sensitivity and specificity for lesser degrees of HE is less established, particularly in MHE. Depending on the set EEG spectral thresholds, sensitivity and specificity varied. In a recent study by Singh and colleagues,[71] with a conventional cutoff theta relative power greater than 35%, sensitivity was 60% and specificity 98%, and accuracy of 79% for diagnosing patients with MHE. In the same study, with a theta relative power of 26.7%, spectral EEG had a sensitivity of 96% and specificity of 84%. In a study by Jackson and colleagues,[72] Short Epoch Dominant Activity Cluster Analysis, which is a more advanced technique for spectral analysis of EEG, was found to have a sensitivity was 74.5% and specificity was 79.4% for any degree of HE with a relative theta power of 22.7.

Unlike the PHES, which is a test battery consisting of 5 pencil and paper tests, EEG is not affected by age, sex, intelligence, education, or ethnicity.[73] EEG also does not require patient cooperation; therefore, it can be performed whether the patient is conscious or in a coma.[60] EEG also can be used to assess the treatment response in patients with cirrhosis with MHE.[72] In the study performed by Singh and colleagues,[71] EEG was able to detect improvements in MDF, and significant changes in alpha, theta, and delta relative power in patients with MHE treated with lactulose.

Current practice guidelines by the AASLD and EASL from 2014 suggest EEG is a complementary neurophysiological test to diagnose MHE and covert HE.[1] EEG itself must be carefully interpreted because findings in HE can be seen in renal dysfunction, hyponatremia, or septic encephalopathy.[74] Although sensitivity and specificity vary depending on relative theta power used and modality of interpreting EEG, EEG is a useful test to evaluate HE independent of education, cooperation, and consciousness, and it can provide the ability to assess disease progression and response to treatment.

SUMMARY

Overall, there are a number of laboratory testing modalities that patients with HE can and may undergo when they present clinically. However, although most of these tests offer insight into the pathogenesis of the HE, they do not have much diagnostic utility on their own. This is true for both the blood testing and the imaging studies.[1] Based on the existing data, much of which is explained in this article, the more promising diagnostic testing seems to be the MRS and the EEG. Before they become an integral part of diagnosis, further research on both of these techniques would need to be performed to identify strict criteria and cutoffs for diagnosing HE as well as associated sensitivities and specificities. Without this, their efficacy remains unclear. As of right now, none of the forms of laboratory testing are required to make a diagnosis of HE and, apart from using EEG in patients with possible covert HE, none of them are recommended by the AASLD/EASL.

DISCLOSURE

The authors have nothing to disclose.

REFERENCES

1. Vilstrup H, et al. Hepatic encephalopathy in chronic liver disease: 2014 practice guideline by the American Association for the Study of Liver Diseases and the European Association for the Study of the Liver. Hepatology 2014;60(2):715–35.
2. Ge PS, Runyon BA. Serum ammonia level for the evaluation of hepatic encephalopathy. JAMA 2014;312(6):643–4.
3. Wong RJ, Gish RG, Ahmed A. Hepatic encephalopathy is associated with significantly increased mortality among patients awaiting liver transplantation. Liver Transpl 2014;20(12):1454–61.
4. Lemberg A, Fernandez MA. Hepatic encephalopathy, ammonia, glutamate, glutamine and oxidative stress. Ann Hepatol 2009;8(2):95–102.
5. Nicolao F, et al. Role of determination of partial pressure of ammonia in cirrhotic patients with and without hepatic encephalopathy. J Hepatol 2003;38(4):441–6.
6. Elgouhari HM, O'Shea R. What is the utility of measuring the serum ammonia level in patients with altered mental status? Cleve Clin J Med 2009;76(4):252–4.
7. Montoliu C, et al. 3-nitro-tyrosine as a peripheral biomarker of minimal hepatic encephalopathy in patients with liver cirrhosis. Am J Gastroenterol 2011;106(9): 1629–37.

8. Rahimi RS, et al. Lactulose vs polyethylene glycol 3350–electrolyte solution for treatment of overt hepatic encephalopathy: the HELP randomized clinical trial. JAMA Intern Med 2014;174(11):1727–33.

9. Bernthal P, et al. Cerebral CT scan abnormalities in cholestatic and hepatocellular disease and their relationship to neuropsychologic test performance. Hepatology 1987;7(1):107–14.

10. Rahimi RS, Rockey DC. Overuse of head computed tomography in cirrhosis with altered mental status. Am J Med Sci 2016;351(5):459–66.

11. Kumar S, et al. A head CT is unnecessary in the initial evaluation of a cirrhotic patient with recurrent hepatic encephalopathy. Ann Hepatol 2018;17(5):810–4.

12. Liotta EM, et al. Osmotic shifts, cerebral edema, and neurologic deterioration in severe hepatic encephalopathy. Crit Care Med 2018;46(2):280–9.

13. Liotta EM, et al. 23.4% saline decreases brain tissue volume in severe hepatic encephalopathy as assessed by a quantitative CT marker. Crit Care Med 2016; 44(1):171–9.

14. Edula RG, Pyrsopoulos NT. New methods of testing and brain imaging in hepatic encephalopathy: a review. Clin Liver Dis 2015;19(3):449–59.

15. Weissenborn K, et al. Functional imaging of the brain in patients with liver cirrhosis. Metab Brain Dis 2004;19(3–4):269–80.

16. Weissenborn K, et al. Correlations between magnetic resonance spectroscopy alterations and cerebral ammonia and glucose metabolism in cirrhotic patients with and without hepatic encephalopathy. Gut 2007;56(12):1736–42.

17. Iversen P, et al. Low cerebral oxygen consumption and blood flow in patients with cirrhosis and an acute episode of hepatic encephalopathy. Gastroenterology 2009;136(3):863–71.

18. Lockwood AH, et al. Altered cerebral blood flow and glucose metabolism in patients with liver disease and minimal encephalopathy. J Cereb Blood Flow Metab 1991;11(2):331–6.

19. Sunil HV, et al. Brain perfusion single photon emission computed tomography abnormalities in patients with minimal hepatic encephalopathy. J Clin Exp Hepatol 2012;2(2):116–21.

20. Nakagawa Y, et al. Single photon emission computed tomography and statistical parametric mapping analysis in cirrhotic patients with and without minimal hepatic encephalopathy. Ann Nucl Med 2004;18(2):123–9.

21. Hauser RA, et al. Blood manganese correlates with brain magnetic resonance imaging changes in patients with liver disease. Can J Neurol Sci 1996;23(2):95–8.

22. Spahr L, et al. Increased blood manganese in cirrhotic patients: relationship to pallidal magnetic resonance signal hyperintensity and neurological symptoms. Hepatology 1996;24(5):1116–20.

23. Maeda H, et al. Brain MR imaging in patients with hepatic cirrhosis: relationship between high intensity signal in basal ganglia on T1-weighted images and elemental concentrations in brain. Neuroradiology 1997;39(8):546–50.

24. Taylor-Robinson SD, et al. MR imaging of the basal ganglia in chronic liver disease: correlation of T1-weighted and magnetisation transfer contrast measurements with liver dysfunction and neuropsychiatric status. Metab Brain Dis 1995;10(2):175–88.

25. Krieger S, et al. MRI findings in chronic hepatic encephalopathy depend on portosystemic shunt: results of a controlled prospective clinical investigation. J Hepatol 1997;27(1):121–6.

26. Butterworth RF. Pathogenesis of hepatic encephalopathy in cirrhosis: the concept of synergism revisited. Metab Brain Dis 2016;31(6):1211–5.

27. Skehan S, et al. Brain MRI changes in chronic liver disease. Eur Radiol 1997;7(6): 905–9.

28. Thuluvath PJ, et al. Increased signals seen in globus pallidus in T1-weighted magnetic resonance imaging in cirrhotics are not suggestive of chronic hepatic encephalopathy. Hepatology 1995;21(2):440–2.

29. Nolte W, et al. Bright basal ganglia in T1-weighted magnetic resonance images are frequent in patients with portal vein thrombosis without liver cirrhosis and not suggestive of hepatic encephalopathy. J Hepatol 1998;29(3):443–9.

30. Fukuzawa T, et al. Magnetic resonance images of the globus pallidus in patients with idiopathic portal hypertension: a quantitative analysis of the relationship between signal intensity and the grade of portosystemic shunt. J Gastroenterol Hepatol 2006;21(5):902–7.

31. Cordoba J, et al. T2 hyperintensity along the cortico-spinal tract in cirrhosis relates to functional abnormalities. Hepatology 2003;38(4):1026–33.

32. Patel N, et al. Changes in brain size in hepatic encephalopathy: a coregistered MRI study. Metab Brain Dis 2004;19(3–4):431–45.

33. Gawne-Cain ML, et al. Fast FLAIR of the brain: the range of appearances in normal subjects and its application to quantification of white-matter disease. Neuroradiology 1997;39(4):243–9.

34. de Leeuw FE, et al. Prevalence of cerebral white matter lesions in elderly people: a population based magnetic resonance imaging study. The Rotterdam Scan Study. J Neurol Neurosurg Psychiatry 2001;70(1):9–14.

35. Rovira A, et al. Decreased white matter lesion volume and improved cognitive function after liver transplantation. Hepatology 2007;46(5):1485–90.

36. Sugimoto R, et al. Value of the apparent diffusion coefficient for quantification of low-grade hepatic encephalopathy. Am J Gastroenterol 2008;103(6):1413–20.

37. Lodi R, et al. Diffusion MRI shows increased water apparent diffusion coefficient in the brains of cirrhotics. Neurology 2004;62(5):762–6.

38. Kale RA, et al. Demonstration of interstitial cerebral edema with diffusion tensor MR imaging in type C hepatic encephalopathy. Hepatology 2006;43(4):698–706.

39. Ranjan P, et al. Cytotoxic edema is responsible for raised intracranial pressure in fulminant hepatic failure: in vivo demonstration using diffusion-weighted MRI in human subjects. Metab Brain Dis 2005;20(3):181–92.

40. Rai V, et al. Measurement of cytotoxic and interstitial components of cerebral edema in acute hepatic failure by diffusion tensor imaging. J Magn Reson Imaging 2008;28(2):334–41.

41. Butterworth RF, et al. Ammonia: key factor in the pathogenesis of hepatic encephalopathy. Neurochem Pathol 1987;6(1–2):1–12.

42. Albrecht J, Faff L. Astrocyte-neuron interactions in hyperammonemia and hepatic encephalopathy. Adv Exp Med Biol 1994;368:45–54.

43. Cordoba J, et al. 1H magnetic resonance in the study of hepatic encephalopathy in humans. Metab Brain Dis 2002;17(4):415–29.

44. Cordoba J, et al. The development of low-grade cerebral edema in cirrhosis is supported by the evolution of (1)H-magnetic resonance abnormalities after liver transplantation. J Hepatol 2001;35(5):598–604.

45. Rovira A, et al. Magnetization transfer ratio values and proton MR spectroscopy of normal-appearing cerebral white matter in patients with liver cirrhosis. AJNR Am J Neuroradiol 2001;22(6):1137–42.

46. Miese F, et al. 1H-MR spectroscopy, magnetization transfer, and diffusion-weighted imaging in alcoholic and nonalcoholic patients with cirrhosis with hepatic encephalopathy. AJNR Am J Neuroradiol 2006;27(5):1019–26.

47. Miese FR, et al. Voxel-based analyses of magnetization transfer imaging of the brain in hepatic encephalopathy. World J Gastroenterol 2009;15(41):5157–64.

48. Goel A, et al. Cerebral oedema in minimal hepatic encephalopathy due to extra-hepatic portal venous obstruction. Liver Int 2010;30(8):1143–51.

49. Balata S, et al. Induced hyperammonemia alters neuropsychology, brain MR spectroscopy and magnetization transfer in cirrhosis. Hepatology 2003;37(4):931–9.

50. Rai R, et al. Reversal of low-grade cerebral edema after lactulose/rifaximin therapy in patients with cirrhosis and minimal hepatic encephalopathy. Clin Transl Gastroenterol 2015;6:e111.

51. Zafiris O, et al. Neural mechanism underlying impaired visual judgement in the dysmetabolic brain: an fMRI study. Neuroimage 2004;22(2):541–52.

52. Zhang LJ, et al. Neural mechanism of cognitive control impairment in patients with hepatic cirrhosis: a functional magnetic resonance imaging study. Acta Radiol 2007;48(5):577–87.

53. Zhong WJ, et al. Abnormal spontaneous brain activity in minimal hepatic encephalopathy: resting-state fMRI study. Diagn Interv Radiol 2016;22(2):196–200.

54. Chen HJ, et al. Aberrant salience network and its functional coupling with default and executive networks in minimal hepatic encephalopathy: a resting-state fMRI study. Sci Rep 2016;6:27092.

55. Manias KA, Peet A. What is MR spectroscopy? Arch Dis Child Educ Pract Ed 2018;103(4):213–6.

56. McPhail MJ, Patel NR, Taylor-Robinson SD. Brain imaging and hepatic encephalopathy. Clin Liver Dis 2012;16(1):57–72.

57. Chavarria L, Cordoba J. Magnetic resonance imaging and spectroscopy in hepatic encephalopathy. J Clin Exp Hepatol 2015;5(Suppl 1):S69–74.

58. Binesh N, et al. Hepatic encephalopathy: a neurochemical, neuroanatomical, and neuropsychological study. J Appl Clin Med Phys 2006;7(1):86–96.

59. Albrecht J, Norenberg MD. Glutamine: a Trojan horse in ammonia neurotoxicity. Hepatology 2006;44(4):788–94.

60. Amodio P, Montagnese S. Clinical neurophysiology of hepatic encephalopathy. J Clin Exp Hepatol 2015;5(Suppl 1):S60–8.

61. Foley JM, Watson CW, Adams RD. Significance of the electroencephalographic changes in hepatic coma. Trans Am Neurol Assoc 1950;51:161–5.

62. Stewart J, et al. Frontal electroencephalogram variables are associated with the outcome and stage of hepatic encephalopathy in acute liver failure. Liver Transpl 2014;20(10):1256–65.

63. Amodio P, et al. Prevalence and prognostic value of quantified electroencephalogram (EEG) alterations in cirrhotic patients. J Hepatol 2001;35(1):37–45.

64. Morgan MY, et al. Qualifying and quantifying minimal hepatic encephalopathy. Metab Brain Dis 2016;31(6):1217–29.

65. Montagnese S, et al. Prognostic benefit of the addition of a quantitative index of hepatic encephalopathy to the MELD score: the MELD-EEG. Liver Int 2015;35(1):58–64.

66. Olesen SS, et al. Electroencephalogram variability in patients with cirrhosis associates with the presence and severity of hepatic encephalopathy. J Hepatol 2016;65(3):517–23.

67. Rehnstrom S, et al. Chronic hepatic encephalopathy. A psychometrical study. Scand J Gastroenterol 1977;12(3):305–11.

68. Weissenborn K, et al. Neurophysiological assessment of early hepatic encephalopathy. Electroencephalogr Clin Neurophysiol 1990;75(4):289–95.

69. Parsons-Smith BG, et al. The electroencephalograph in liver disease. Lancet 1957;273(7001):867–71.
70. Van der Rijt CC, et al. Objective measurement of hepatic encephalopathy by means of automated EEG analysis. Electroencephalogr Clin Neurophysiol 1984;57(5):423–6.
71. Singh J, et al. Spectral electroencephalogram in liver cirrhosis with minimal hepatic encephalopathy before and after lactulose therapy. J Gastroenterol Hepatol 2016;31(6):1203–9.
72. Jackson CD, et al. New spectral thresholds improve the utility of the electroencephalogram for the diagnosis of hepatic encephalopathy. Clin Neurophysiol 2016;127(8):2933–41.
73. Campagna F, et al. Confounders in the detection of minimal hepatic encephalopathy: a neuropsychological and quantified EEG study. Liver Int 2015;35(5): 1524–32.
74. Ferenci P. Hepatic encephalopathy. Gastroenterol Rep (Oxf) 2017;5(2):138–47.

Minimal Hepatic Encephalopathy

Briette Verken Karanfilian, MD[a,1], Taeyang Park, MD[a,*], Frank Senatore, MD[b],
Vinod K. Rustgi, MD, MBA[c]

KEYWORDS

- Minimal hepatic encephalopathy • Subclinical hepatic encephalopathy
- West Haven criteria • Medical apps • EncephalApp • Patient buddy app
- Stroop test

KEY POINTS

- Minimal hepatic encephalopathy, previously referred to as subclinical hepatic encephalopathy, represents the earliest and mildest form of hepatic encephalopathy.
- There is no gold standard for diagnosing minimal hepatic encephalopathy; however, a number of validated testing modalities have been devised to detect this neurocognitive complication.
- New technologies have allowed for the development of medically related apps that can be used to diagnose and monitor minimal hepatic encephalopathy.
- Early detection has become paramount with the discovery of an association with worse clinical outcomes in patients diagnosed with minimal hepatic encephalopathy.

INTRODUCTION

Hepatic encephalopathy (HE) is one of the many sequelae of decompensated liver disease. It consists of a potentially reversible spectrum of neurologic and psychiatric manifestations that can range from subclinical alteration in mental status to coma. Originally, the main classification system used to define the continuum of HE was the West Haven Criteria, which classifies patients' disease into 1 of 5 categories, with less severe manifestations qualifying as either minimal or grade I disease.[1] The West Haven Criteria were used for many years, but in 2011, the International Society for Hepatic Encephalopathy and Nitrogen Metabolism created a newer, less subjective grading system that classifies HE as either covert or overt based on symptoms

[a] Department of Internal Medicine, Rutgers- Robert Wood Johnson Medical School, 125 Paterson Street, CAB 7302, New Brunswick, NJ 08901, USA; [b] Department of Gastroenterology and Hepatology, Rutgers- Robert Wood Johnson Medical School, 125 Paterson Street, CAB 7302, New Brunswick, NJ 08901, USA; [c] Center for Liver Diseases and Masses, Robert Wood Johnson Medical School, Clinical Academic Building (CAB), 125 Paterson Street, Suite 5100B, New Brunswick, NJ 08901, USA
[1] Present address: 110 Somerset Street, Apartment #2203, New Brunswick, NJ 08901.
* Corresponding author.
E-mail address: drsun0513@gmail.com

Clin Liver Dis 24 (2020) 209–218
https://doi.org/10.1016/j.cld.2020.01.012
1089-3261/20/© 2020 Elsevier Inc. All rights reserved.

liver.theclinics.com

and suggested operative criteria. The International Society for Hepatic Encephalopathy and Nitrogen Metabolism category of covert HE, or clinically undetectable HE, encompasses both the West Haven Criteria's categories of minimal and grade I disease. The patients who fall into these categories are those with minimal HE (MHE).

MHE, previously referred to as subclinical HE, represents the earliest and mildest form of HE.[2] More significantly, it is the most under-recognized and underdiagnosed form of HE. Patients with MHE do not exhibit any clinical evidence of cognitive changes, but rather have slow alterations in their psychomotor or neuropsychiatric functioning.[3] It is estimated that as many as 80% of patients with chronic liver disease suffer from MHE.[4] Currently, there is no gold standard for diagnosing MHE; however, a number of validated testing modalities have been devised to detect this neurocognitive complication.[5,6] Some of these testing modalities created to diagnose MHE can also prognosticate those who are at risk for progressing to overt HE.[3]

Although the recognition of MHE can be quite challenging, the emphasis on early detection has become paramount with the discovery of an association with worse clinical outcomes in patients diagnosed with MHE. Patients with MHE are at a higher risk for hospitalization and motor vehicle collisions.[4,7] Even more, individuals with MHE are at a higher risk of progressing to overt HE, have impaired quality of life, and have an increase in overall mortality rates.[4,8]

The push for developing newer tools in the diagnosis of MHE surrounds the concept that HE leads to prolonged hospitalizations and billions of dollars for our health care system. At the same time, MHE by itself does not require hospitalization or emergent medical care, affording this entity to become a target for management approaches if appropriately diagnosed early in its course. In actuality, targeting the diagnosis of MHE is a preventative method with the potential for enormous cost savings and improved long-term clinical outcomes for patients with chronic liver disease. Early recognition of MHE can potentially decrease the socioeconomic burden associated with this disease and improve quality of life for these patients.[9]

PSYCHOMETRIC HEPATIC ENCEPHALOPATHY SCORE

The Psychometric Hepatic Encephalopathy Score (PHES), also referred to as the Portosystemic Encephalopathy Syndrome Test, consists of a series of tests that evaluate cognitive and psychomotor processing speed and visuomotor coordination. The score was first developed and standardized in Germany. Later, the Hepatic Encephalopathy Consensus Group at the World Congress of Gastroenterology in 1998 recognized the PHES as the gold standard for the diagnosis of MHE. The test has gained popularity as it is easily administered in 10 to 20 minutes without professionally trained personnel or advanced equipment.[9]

The PHES consists of 5 paper-and-pencil psychometric tests: the digit symbol test, line tracing test, number connections tests A and B, and serial dotting test. Each test is scored based on standard deviations (Z-scores) from average scores of healthy controls. A patient's final score can range from −18 to +6 points. The diagnostic threshold distinguishing a positive result for MHE is a score of less than −4. The sensitivity and specificity of PHES is 96% and 100%, respectively.[6]

The PHES has also been used as a prognostic tool. Patients who received a score consistent with MHE were shown to have a higher probability of developing overt HE compared with those who were not diagnosed with MHE.[8] Recently, a study looked at the association between the PHES and the Psychomotor Vigilance Task, which is a widely used tool to assess vigilance and driving ability. The study showed that those with a pathologic PHES had worse Psychomotor Vigilance Task indices compared with those with normal PHES.[10] This association expands on the usefulness of the PHES as a prognostic tool specific to certain activities of daily living for patients.

Nevertheless, the PHES is not without limitations. Although the test does not require prior training or equipment to conduct, the 10 to 20 minutes required to complete it is time consuming. In an era in the United States where the average office visit follow-up appointment is 15 minutes, combined with escalating financial challenges within the health care system, the role of a 10- to 20-minute test becomes very limited. As well, there is no additional reimbursement for administering the PHES, which is an unfortunate but real factor to consider when managing patients with chronic liver disease. The PHES can also be influenced by many factors, including age and the level of education of the test taker.[9]

In 2011, Riggio and colleagues[11] investigated potential solutions to the time limitation of the PHES. They conducted a study showing that a lower number of subtests within the PHES can identify patients with MHE without decreasing diagnostic accuracy. They referred to this abbreviated version of the PHES as the Simplified PHES, which only includes the digit symbol test, serial dotting test, and line tracing test. Using the Simplified PHES offers a modest decrease of about 40% in the time required for MHE screening.

REPEATABLE BATTERY FOR THE ASSESSMENT OF NEUROPSYCHOLOGICAL STATUS

The Repeatable Battery for the Assessment of Neuropsychological Status (RBANS) test is also a paper-and-pencil test, although there are fewer data published regarding this testing modality and it is used less frequently. The RBANS was initially designed to diagnose other neurocognitive disorders, such as schizophrenia and dementia, and was later applied to patients with liver disease to evaluate for MHE. The test evaluates global cognitive functioning in terms of 5 major domains: attention, delayed memory, immediate memory, language, and visuospatial construction. Index scores are converted to age-based standard scores. The International Society for Hepatic Encephalopathy and Nitrogen Metabolism has recommended the use of RBANS to assess patients for HE, especially in the United States because there is population-based standardization and norming. However, as mentioned, the data behind its effectiveness in diagnosing MHE are limited. One study showed its sensitivity in diagnosing covert HE to be as low as 35.3%.[12] This may be due to the fact that 2 of the domains of this testing modality (delayed memory and language), are usually not impaired in MHE.[9] There has yet to be a head-to-head study comparing the efficacy of RBANS to PHES.

INHIBITORY CONTROL TEST

The Inhibitory Control Test (ICT) is one of the more commonly used testing modalities to diagnose MHE. It is a computerized test that is designed to assess attention, response inhibition, and working memory. During the test, patients are shown a series of letters on the computer screen at 500-millisecond intervals. They are instructed to press the space bar every time they are shown alternating letters such as an "X" followed by a "Y or a "Y" followed by "X," which are referred to as "targets." Meanwhile, they are also instructed to ignore what are referred to as "lures," which are pairs of "XX" or "YY." Ideally, patients will respond to all 212 targets, showing intact attention, ignore all 40 lures, showing intact response inhibition, and do so with short reaction times.[8]

It has been shown that overall the ICT has excellent sensitivity and specificity when it comes to diagnosing MHE, although there has been some controversy regarding which ICT parameter is the most useful. For instance, a study conducted in the United States in 2008 postulated that the aspect of the ICT with the highest sensitivity and specificity for diagnosing MHE was incorrect response to lures. The study showed that incorrect response to more than 5 lures correlated with an 88% sensitivity in diagnosing MHE.[13] However, a follow-up study conducted in Italy found that looking at lures alone was not adequate to detect all of the patients with MHE diagnosed by other psychometric testing, such as PHES. Instead, this study found that the ICT scoring with the best sensitivity and specificity for diagnosing MHE was based on lures weighted by target accuracy.[14] The discrepancy between these first 2 studies was likely due to the fact that the patients included in the study in Italy had more advanced disease and a lower level of education.

A more recent comprehensive study evaluated all possible ICT parameters and their accuracy in diagnosing MHE, taking into account patient age and level of education. This study found that focusing on target accuracy alone resulted in the highest sensitivity and specificity for diagnosing MHE.[12] The study suggested that the reason the previous research studies had been inaccurate was that the usefulness of lures and weighted lures is actually heavily influenced by patient age and level of education. Therefore, although this newer study found that the sensitivity for lures alone was 82%, similar to what had been previously published, it also found that the specificity of lures alone was only 36%. Additionally, this newer study also showed that weighted lures were only associated with a sensitivity of 41%. These values paled in comparison to the sensitivity and specificity for target accuracy, which were 82% and 98%, respectively.[12]

The American Association for the Study of Liver Diseases/European Association for the Study of the Liver practice guidelines support the validity of the ICT. There is excellent test–retest reliability. Additionally, the ICT has been shown to be useful in prognostication of patients developing overt HE and it has been shown to be useful in tracking clinical improvement following treatment of MHE.[13]

CRITICAL FLICKER FREQUENCY

Another testing modality is the Critical Flicker Frequency (CFF) test. During CFF, the patient watches a series of pulses of light, which are initially displayed at such a high frequency that they appear to be a steady stream of light. As the test continues, the frequency of the pulses of light decreases. As soon as the patient notices the light starting to flicker, as opposed to appearing as a steady stream of light, they are supposed to press a button. The patients with MHE will have impaired visual perception and reaction time, so they will not be able to identify the initiation of flickering as quickly as patients without MHE.[15] One study showed that CFF had a sensitivity of 55% and a specificity of 100% for diagnosing MHE when a flicker frequency threshold of 39 Hz was used.[16] A large meta-analysis that included 9 studies found that CFF had a sensitivity of 61% and specificity of 79% in diagnosing MHE.[17] Although this test has fairly high specificity, it has a relatively low sensitivity, which limits its use as a first-line test.

Despite this finding, one of the main advantages of CFF is that results are not influenced by patient age or patient education level.[18] Furthermore, when combined with Child-Pugh class, CFF results have been shown to have prognostic value in predicting development of overt HE.[19] Repeat CFF testing after treatment with lactulose has been used successfully to assess recovery of patients.[20]

SCAN PACKAGE

The Scan Package is another computerized test assessing reaction time to visual stimuli. It is composed of 3 parts. The first part is the Simple Reaction Time test, during which a visual stimulus is flashed on the computer screen and the patient is supposed to respond by pressing the space bar on the keyboard when they see the stimulus. The second part is slightly more complex, and it is referred to as the Choice Reaction Time test. During this section, either the number 1 or the number 3 is displayed on the computer screen, and the patient must press the appropriate corresponding number on the computer keyboard. Last, there is the Scan Reaction Time test, during which 36 pairs of numbers are shown and the subject has to respond by pressing 1 if there are pairs in common or 3 if there are no pairs in common. The total number of stimuli that the patient responds to is calculated as a percent to determine their accuracy. Additionally, accuracy-adjusted reaction times are also calculated. A patient's final result is calculated as a Z-score that is corrected for age and level of education. One study has shown that patients with a history of overt HE performed worse on the Scan Package test than those who never had overt HE.[21]

CONTINUOUS REACTION TIME TEST

Whereas the CFF and Scan Package evaluate patients' reaction time to visual stimuli, the Continuous Reaction Time (CRT) test evaluates their reaction time to auditory stimuli. In this computerized test, a total of 150 auditory stimuli are played over a period of 10 minutes. The sounds occur at random intervals ranging from 2 to 6 seconds in length. Each time the patient hears a sound, they are supposed to press a button. The test analyzes patients' reaction speed, attention, and inhibitory control.[22] Patients' results are reported in terms of a CRT index, which is calculated as 50 percentile/(90–10 percentile). The index measures the consistency of the patient's reaction times. The higher the CRT index, the more consistent the patient was in pressing the button at the appropriate times. CRT index values greater than or equal to 1.9 are considered normal. CRT index values less than 1.9 are diagnostic of MHE. This testing modality is commonly used in Denmark. Similar to the CFF, the CRT test results are not influenced by patient age or level of education.

THE ELECTROENCEPHALOGRAM

Electroencephalogram (EEG) has been used for a long time to diagnose HE. In the 1950s, monomorphic slow waves were first observed in the frontal regions of EEG in patients with covert HE.[23] Subsequent observations showed gradual slowing in the EEG activity from alpha range (8–13 Hz) toward theta (4–7 Hz) and delta (1–4 Hz) to eventually isoelectric readings with advancing stages of HE.[24]

One disadvantage of EEG is that its interpretation is operator dependent and may not produce adequate replicability. Spectral analysis of EEG has been proposed to provide more objective analysis but its effectiveness in diagnosing minimal encephalopathy has been questioned.[9] A study by Amodio and colleagues[24] showed there was no statistically significant difference in accuracy of spectral EEG analysis compared with that of qualitative visual EEG readings or semiquantitative visual assessment.[22] Nonetheless, the study concluded that spectral EEG analysis may reduce operator dependability and may improve assessment of mild encephalopathy. Another study using spectral analysis during sleep showed that mean dominant frequency changes during sleep are an early marker of cerebral dysfunction in cirrhotic patients with MHE.[25]

Recently, there have been more advanced developments to apply EEG in assessing those with HE. In one study, to produce more objective results, the artificial neural network expert system based interpretation was used and it was shown to be a useful tool to establish objective staging of HE in patients with cirrhosis (Pellegrini 2005).

Another study applied a system for spatiotemporal decomposition SEDACA (short epoch, dominant activity, cluster analysis) in analyzing EEG of cirrhotic patients. The study found that applying SEDACA produced potentially more diagnostic information than conventional analyzing technique, which allowed further differentiating patients with MHE from healthy individuals.[26]

The EEG is undoubtedly a reliable and objective means of diagnosing HE. Further advantages include that its results are independent of age and level of education. Furthermore, it has also shown prognostic value for the development of HE and mortality in cirrhotic patients.[27]

APPS

Strategies testing for cognitive dysfunction are challenging and not easily implemented nor routinely practiced in the medical community. There are certain universal limitations for all of the aforementioned diagnostic modalities in detecting MHE (**Table 1**). The time required to administer these tests stands as the focal weakness. This has paved the way for the development of new tools that use technology to deliver reliable results in a streamlined fashion. Technology allows for shorter methods of diagnosis that are easily accessible, reliable, and applicable.

In an age of smartphones and tablet devices, apps have opened the door as a new avenue in which the medical community can assimilate with their patients to deliver high quality care. Apps can range in terms of their cost to develop, but their accessibility and streamlined complexity make the cost–benefit continuum frequently lean in the positive direction.

The Stroop Test is a novel assessment tool published in 2013 testing mental speed and flexibility to diagnose MHE.[28] Its assessment relies on 2 separate variables. First, the patient has to identify the color of the text of words written on a screen. Second, the patient has to identify the color of the text of words again, but this time the words themselves are actual colors different from the text color. These tests are compared and are standardized based on several simple patient demographics. It

Table 1
Diagnostic tests for MHE

Name	Sensitivity (%)	Specificity (%)	Ease of Use	Time Requirement
PHES	90	100	1	3
Simplified PHES[11]	90	100	1	2
RBANS[12,33]	35	100	2	3
ICT – 5 Lures	82	36	2	2
ICT – Lures adjusted for age and education	18	98		
ICT – Weight Lures	41	99		
ICT – Targets[12]	82	98		
CFF	61	79	2	2
CRT[22,30]	93	92	2	2
EEG[34]	60	98	3	3
Scan Package[35]	No data	No data	2	3
Stroop Test	78	90	1	1

Ease of use: 1 (easy); 2 (requires training or equipment), and 3 (requires training and equipment). Time requirement: 1 (<5 min), 2 (5–15 min), or 3 (>15 min).

is administered in less than 5 minutes and is extremely easy to use, requiring no training or repetitive use to master. The results are automatically calculated and provided on a report that is simple to interpret.

The first data supporting this app came from a study comparing 124 patients with cirrhosis with 134 controls. The PHES and ICT were used to compare against the Stroop Test. The Stroop Test was able to predict patients who had a prior episode of overt HE and was statistically significant ($P<.0001$) at distinguishing patients with MHE compared with those without MHE.[28] The sensitivity and specificity of the Stroop Test were 78% and 90%, respectively.[28] A follow-up validation study comparing 167 patients with cirrhosis compared with 114 controls showed the Stroop Test to have good face validity, test–retest reliability and external validity.[29]

This platform was then expanded in a multicenter study at 4 centers in the United States: Virginia Commonwealth University, McGuire VA Medical Center, Cleveland Clinic, and University of Arkansas for Medical Sciences.[30] This study evaluated 437 cirrhotics against 308 controls and demonstrated good sensitivity for diagnosing MHE and predictive capability for the development of overt HE.[30]

The success of the Stroop Test led to the development of the first mobile app with the intentions of improving the diagnostic accuracy and efficiency of MHE. The Stroop Test was integrated into the EncephalApp, which is a free app available through the app store of all Android and Apple iOS devices. The accessibility of technology is demonstrated first hand in this product, because it has rapidly expanded in popularity throughout the world and is now available in English, Spanish, German, Indonesian, Romanian, Slovakian, Thai, and Mandarin. To date, this is the most successful and well-studied app conceived for the detection of MHE.

Given the multitude of diagnostic tests that have been investigated to diagnosis MHE, a recent study evaluated the role of using single versus combination testing. This multicenter study included 437 patients at 3 centers. **Table 2** shows the prevalence of MHE,[31] with the Stroop Test showing greater sensitivity in predicting MHE. Overall, the PHES or the Stroop alone or the PHES combined with Stroop Testing were equivalent to diagnose MHE and predict overt HE.[31]

An app targeted for patients on a more global health care level has been developed, with implications related to MHE. The Patient Buddy App was developed to facilitate communication and educate patients and their care managers. As well, it is intended to remove many postdischarge barriers that exist after a patient's hospitalization.

Specifically, the Patient Buddy App assists patients in understanding discharge instructions, improving patient communication of new or recurrent symptoms, reinforcing prescription directions, setting follow-up reminders, reporting medical side effects, and answering caregiver questions. This app has the ability to send automatic alerts for critical values and adherence concerns. It requires a fee-based subscription

Table 2 Prevalence of MHE	
Test	**Prevalence (%)**
PHES + ICT	18
PHES + Stroop	25
ICT + Stroop	29
ICT	35
PHES	37
Stroop	54

purchased by medical practices and health care organizations to give to their patients with the intention of improving quality outcomes and net cost burden.

The Patient Buddy App has been shown to prevent HE-related readmissions by tracking variables specific to this neurocognitive complication. In a proof-of-concept pilot study, 40 cirrhotic patients were followed for 30 days after discharge, along with 40 caregivers.[32] Seventeen of the cirrhotic patients were readmitted within 30 days, none of which were related to HE. Eight potential HE-related admissions were prevented using this app.[32] Overall, this study showed the feasibility of the Patient Buddy App and its applicability to patients with chronic liver disease.

This app allows care managers to monitor medication adherence, daily sodium intake, and weights among other variables. Medication noncompliance is one of the most common causes for neurocognitive decompensation in patients with chronic liver disease. If recognized early, interventions can be made to prevent further progression from minimal to overt HE, avoiding more catastrophic complications for patients and higher cost burden for care managers. Even more, the Patient Buddy App has the EncephalApp Stroop Test incorporated into its section monitoring HE.[32] This allows the care manager to have their patient perform daily MHE evaluations and track small changes that can predict slight changes in neurocognition.

Technology in the form of medically related apps is likely to continue to expand over the next decade, providing global accessibility and the potential to transform health care. MHE is just one of many diagnoses that can be targeted to deliver better quality care. To date, the Stroop Test and PHES are the most efficacious tools available to identify MHE and predict progression to overt HE.

DISCLOSURE

The authors have nothing to disclose.

REFERENCES

1. Dharel N, Bajaj JS. Definition and nomenclature of hepatic encephalopathy. J Clin Exp Hepatol 2015;5(Suppl 1):S37–41.
2. Amodio P, et al. Characteristics of minimal hepatic encephalopathy. Metab Brain Dis 2004;19(3–4):253–67.
3. Vilstrup H, et al. Hepatic encephalopathy in chronic liver disease: 2014 practice guideline by the American Association for the Study of Liver Diseases and the European Association for the Study of the Liver. Hepatology 2014;60(2):715–35.
4. Ridola L, Cardinale V, Riggio O. The burden of minimal hepatic encephalopathy: from diagnosis to therapeutic strategies. Ann Gastroenterol 2018;31(2):151–64.
5. Lauridsen MM, Schaffalitzky de Muckadell OB, Vilstrup H. Minimal hepatic encephalopathy characterized by parallel use of the continuous reaction time and portosystemic encephalopathy tests. Metab Brain Dis 2015;30(5):1187–92.
6. Weissenborn K. Diagnosis of minimal hepatic encephalopathy. J Clin Exp Hepatol 2015;5(Suppl 1):S54–9.
7. Bajaj JS, et al. Minimal hepatic encephalopathy is associated with motor vehicle crashes: the reality beyond the driving test. Hepatology 2009;50(4):1175–83.
8. Tapper EB, et al. Diagnosis of minimal hepatic encephalopathy: a systematic review of point-of-care diagnostic tests. Am J Gastroenterol 2018;113(4):529–38.
9. Nabi E, Bajaj JS. Useful tests for hepatic encephalopathy in clinical practice. Curr Gastroenterol Rep 2014;16(1):362.

10. Formentin C, et al. The psychomotor vigilance task: role in the diagnosis of hepatic encephalopathy and relationship with driving ability. J Hepatol 2019;70(4): 648–57.
11. Riggio O, et al. A simplified psychometric evaluation for the diagnosis of minimal hepatic encephalopathy. Clin Gastroenterol Hepatol 2011;9(7):613–6.e1.
12. Goldbecker A, et al. Comparison of the most favoured methods for the diagnosis of hepatic encephalopathy in liver transplantation candidates. Gut 2013;62(10): 1497–504.
13. Bajaj JS, et al. Inhibitory control test for the diagnosis of minimal hepatic encephalopathy. Gastroenterology 2008;135(5):1591–600.e1.
14. Amodio P, et al. Improving the inhibitory control task to detect minimal hepatic encephalopathy. Gastroenterology 2010;139(2):510–8, 518.e1-2.
15. Dhiman RK, et al. Diagnosis and prognostic significance of minimal hepatic encephalopathy in patients with cirrhosis of liver. Dig Dis Sci 2010;55(8):2381–90.
16. Kircheis G, Hilger N, Haussinger D. Value of critical flicker frequency and psychometric hepatic encephalopathy score in diagnosis of low-grade hepatic encephalopathy. Gastroenterology 2014;146(4):961–9.
17. Torlot FJ, McPhail MJ, Taylor-Robinson SD. Meta-analysis: the diagnostic accuracy of critical flicker frequency in minimal hepatic encephalopathy. Aliment Pharmacol Ther 2013;37(5):527–36.
18. Kircheis G, et al. Hepatic encephalopathy and fitness to drive. Gastroenterology 2009;137(5):1706–15.e1-9.
19. Romero-Gomez M, et al. Value of the critical flicker frequency in patients with minimal hepatic encephalopathy. Hepatology 2007;45(4):879–85.
20. Sharma P, Sharma BC, Sarin SK. Prevalence of abnormal psychometric tests and critical flicker frequency after clinical recovery of overt hepatic encephalopathy. Neurol India 2010;58(2):220–4.
21. Sakamoto M, et al. Assessment and usefulness of clinical scales for semiquantification of overt hepatic encephalopathy. Clin Liver Dis 2012;16(1):27–42.
22. Lauridsen MM, et al. The continuous reaction times method for diagnosing, grading, and monitoring minimal/covert hepatic encephalopathy. Metab Brain Dis 2013;28(2):231–4.
23. Foley JM, Watson CW, Adams RD. Significance of the electroencephalographic changes in hepatic coma. Trans Am Neurol Assoc 1950;51:161–5.
24. Amodio P, et al. Prevalence and prognostic value of quantified electroencephalogram (EEG) alterations in cirrhotic patients. J Hepatol 2001;35(1):37–45.
25. Martino ME, et al. Sleep electroencephalogram alterations disclose initial stage of encephalopathy. Methods Find Exp Clin Pharmacol 2002;24(Suppl D):119–22.
26. Montagnese S, Jackson C, Morgan MY. Spatio-temporal decomposition of the electroencephalogram in patients with cirrhosis. J Hepatol 2007;46(3):447–58.
27. Amodio P, et al. Spectral versus visual EEG analysis in mild hepatic encephalopathy. Clin Neurophysiol 1999;110(8):1334–44.
28. Bajaj JS, et al. The Stroop smartphone application is a short and valid method to screen for minimal hepatic encephalopathy. Hepatology 2013;58(3):1122–32.
29. Bajaj JS, et al. Validation of EncephalApp, smartphone-based Stroop test, for the diagnosis of covert hepatic encephalopathy. Clin Gastroenterol Hepatol 2015; 13(10):1828–35.e1.
30. Allampati S, et al. Diagnosis of minimal hepatic encephalopathy using Stroop EncephalApp: a multicenter US-based, norm-based study. Am J Gastroenterol 2016;111(1):78–86.

31. Duarte-Rojo A, Allampati S, Thacker LR, et al. Diagnosis of covert hepatic encephalopathy: a multi-center study testing the utility of single versus combined testing. Metab Brain Dis 2018;34(1):289–95.
32. Ganapathy D, et al. The patient buddy app can potentially prevent hepatic encephalopathy-related readmissions. Liver Int 2017;37(12):1843–51.
33. Patidar KR, Bajaj JS. Covert and overt hepatic encephalopathy: diagnosis and management. Clin Gastroenterol Hepatol 2015;13(12):2048–61.
34. Singh J, et al. Spectral electroencephalogram in liver cirrhosis with minimal hepatic encephalopathy before and after lactulose therapy. J Gastroenterol Hepatol 2016;31(6):1203–9.
35. Montagnese S, et al. Simple tools for complex syndromes: a three-level difficulty test for hepatic encephalopathy. Dig Liver Dis 2012;44(11):957–60.

Prognosis of Hepatic Encephalopathy

Anita Krishnarao, MD, MPH[a], Fredric D. Gordon, MD[a,b],*

KEYWORDS

- Encephalopathy • Prognosis • Decompensation • Hospitalization • Survival

KEY POINTS

- Both subclinical and overt hepatic encephalopathy predict a poor prognosis.
- Risk factors for a poor prognosis include acid-base and electrolyte disturbances, diminished renal function, biochemical evidence of poor hepatic synthetic function, and acute-on-chronic liver failure.
- Pre-transplant hepatic encephalopathy may impact post-transplant outcomes and neurocognitive function.
- Treatment of hepatic encephalopathy reduces the risk of recurrence, frequency of hospitalization, hospital costs, and mortality.

INTRODUCTION

The development of hepatic encephalopathy (HE) is one of the markers of decompensated cirrhosis, and the presence of HE has been thought to carry significant prognostic value for several decades. HE was incorporated into early prognostic tools including the Child-Turcotte-Pugh (CTP) score based on clinical experience at the time, and many studies have since demonstrated the association between subclinical or overt HE and worse clinical outcomes including increased falls, increased motor vehicle accidents, more frequent hospitalizations, and worse overall survival. The presence of HE in the pre-transplant setting has also been shown to have prognostic implications after liver transplantation. Although standard HE therapy with rifaximin and lactulose is associated with decreased hospitalizations and mortality in patients with overt HE in the pre-transplant setting, the clinical and prognostic impacts of HE therapy for patients with subclinical HE and for patients in the post-transplant setting have yet to be fully elucidated.

[a] Division of Transplantation and Hepatobiliary Diseases, Lahey Hospital and Medical Center, 41 Mall Road, Burlington, MA 01805, USA; [b] Tufts Medical School, 145 Harrison Avenue, Boston, MA 02111, USA
* Corresponding author. Division of Transplantation and Hepatobiliary Diseases, Lahey Hospital and Medical Center, 41 Mall Road, Burlington, MA 01805.
E-mail address: fredric.d.gordon@lahey.org

Clin Liver Dis 24 (2020) 219–229
https://doi.org/10.1016/j.cld.2020.01.004
1089-3261/20/© 2020 Elsevier Inc. All rights reserved.

liver.theclinics.com

IMPACT AND PROGNOSIS OF SUBCLINICAL HEPATIC ENCEPHALOPATHY

Subclinical HE is defined as neurocognitive dysfunction that can lead to deficits in attention and orientation, which result in learning impairment and loss of working memory.[1] Intelligence IQ and communications skills are generally preserved in subclinical HE, and the diagnosis often requires psychometric testing because of the lack of specific signs or symptoms. Subclinical HE has been shown to be present in as many as 80% of cirrhotic patients in the United States, and associated deficits can predispose patients to impaired quality of life.[2,3] Patients with subclinical HE have been found to have greater impairments in sleep, eating, home management, mobility and driving, self-care, social interaction, and emotional behavior compared to patients with cirrhosis without subclinical HE.[2,4] These deficits may also prevent the constant vigilance and coordination required for many professions. It has therefore been suggested that subclinical HE not only has the potential to endanger patients and coworkers during complex occupational tasks, but it can subsequently affect the socioeconomic status of patients as a result of poor work performance.[5]

Although the presence of subclinical HE may not always be immediately apparent, it has been linked to many relevant clinical outcomes, including increased falls, increased motor vehicle accidents, increased hospitalizations, and worse overall survival. Retrospective data published in 2011 revealed that 40% of cirrhotic patients with subclinical HE had falls compared to 12.9% of cirrhotic patients without subclinical HE who had falls over the study period ($P<.001$), and risk of falls was found to be higher among patients on psychoactive medications such as antidepressant therapy.[6] Prospective data from 2010 also demonstrated that there is a higher risk for motor vehicle accidents in patients with cirrhosis with subclinical HE compared to patients with cirrhosis without subclinical HE (22% vs 7%, $P = .03$), and the rate of accidents in 1 year among those with subclinical HE was shown to be far in excess of the baseline rate of accidents in the populations studied (3%).[7] Patients with subclinical HE have been previously shown to have poor on-road driving test performance also, which is in line with this increased risk of accidents, and this is thought to be related to inherent attention deficits and predisposition to fatigue.[8] Prospective data have also shown that subclinical HE is associated with double the risk of hospitalization compared to cirrhotic patients without subclinical HE, and this increased risk was independent of the underlying model for end-stage liver disease (MELD) score. Cirrhotic patients with subclinical HE were at increased risk for hospitalizations for liver-related and non-liver related diagnoses compared to patients with cirrhosis without subclinical HE.[9]

Patients with subclinical HE also have a higher likelihood of developing overt HE, which carries even greater prognostic significance, and multiple studies have shown that more than 50% of patients with subclinical HE develop an episode of overt HE within a period of 2 weeks to 2 years after the initial diagnosis[10,11] (**Fig. 1**). Specific subgroups that seem to carry this higher risk of progression from subclinical to overt HE are males, those with alcoholic etiology of cirrhosis or lower glutamine levels, and patients with esophageal varices.[12–14] The pathogenesis of why these certain groups are at higher risk for progression to overt HE, however, is poorly understood. Subclinical HE has also independently been shown to be associated with worse survival even in the absence of overt hepatic encephalopathy[15] (**Fig. 2**). Prior studies have suggested that this association of subclinical HE with worse survival is related to the severity of underlying liver disease, but subclinical HE CTP scores have been shown to be independent predictors of poor survival in patients with cirrhosis.[11] The presence of subclinical HE has similarly been associated with an increased risk of death and liver transplantation, and this association was noted to exist independently of MELD

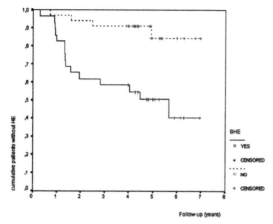

Fig. 1. Cumulative proportion of patients without hepatic encephalopathy (HE) in relation to previous diagnosis of subclinical hepatic encephalopathy (SHE). SHE diagnosis predicts overt HE in follow-up (P<.005). (*From* Romero-Gomez M, Boza F, Garcia-Valdecasas MS, et al. Subclinical hepatic encephalopathy predicts the development of over hepatic encephalopathy. Am J Gastroenterol 2001; 96: 2718-2723; with permission.)

score.[9] It is therefore important to recognize and diagnose subclinical HE, not only as a risk factor for developing overt HE, but also because of its impact on daily functioning and its independent role in determining overall prognosis.

HEPATIC ENCEPHALOPATHY AND SURVIVAL-RELATED OUTCOMES

Although recent data have demonstrated the clinical importance and prognostic significance of subclinical HE, overt HE has been validated as an important marker of

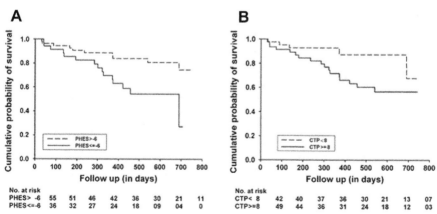

Fig. 2. (*A*) Survival probability of cirrhotic patients, classified into 2 groups according to psychometric hepatic encephalopathy score (PHES) ≤-6 and greater than -6 [$P = .003$, log-rank test (Mantel-Cox)]. (*B*) Survival probability of cirrhotic patients, classified into 2 groups according to CTP score ≥ 8 and <8 [$P = .01$, log-rank test (Mantel-Cox)]. (*From* Dhiman RK, Kurmi R, Thumburu KK, et al. Diagnosis and prognostic significance of minimal hepatic encephalopathy in patients with cirrhosis of liver. Dig Dis Sci 2010; 55: 2381-2390; with permission.)

overall prognosis in cirrhosis for at least the past 20 years. The development of overt HE is one of the events that defines the decompensated phase of liver disease similar to variceal bleeding or the presence of ascites. The prognostic value of HE was initially recognized in the 1960s when HE was adopted as 1 of 5 variables in the Child-Turcotte classification, which was eventually modified to become the CTP score in 1973.[16,17] The CTP score was originally developed to predict survival probabilities among patients with cirrhosis after portocaval shunt surgery, but this score has since been more broadly used to reflect the severity of liver disease. Although the selection of hepatic encephalopathy as a variable was based on clinical experience at the time and not multivariate analysis, patients in different CTP classifications at the time of initial studies did demonstrate statistically significant differences in 3-year and 10-year survival after surgery.[16]

Early data from the 1990s subsequently showed that the development of the first episode of acute HE in cirrhotic patients is independently associated with shorter life expectancies, and the cumulative survival for patients who developed HE was less than 50% at 1 year and less than 25% at 3 years.[18] This survival data were also noted to be worse compared with patients undergoing liver transplantation at that time, which again reflects the importance of HE as a prognostic marker. Multiple follow-up studies have since validated the association of HE with increased hospitalization rates and worse survival. A population-based cohort study of patients with alcoholic cirrhosis from 2010 similarly demonstrated worse 1-year mortality of 64% in patients who developed HE alone compared with a 1-year mortality of 17% in patients who did not develop complications of liver disease. The development of HE in this cohort also had a worse 1-year mortality compared with patients who developed either variceal bleeding or ascites, which suggests that HE may potentially hold more prognostic value than other markers of decompensation.[19]

It has also been proposed that the presence and the duration of an episode of acute HE play prognostic roles in overall survival-related outcomes. Data from a retrospective study in 2018 suggested that the length of time a patient with cirrhosis remains in overt HE during an acute episode (defined as >48 hours) correlates with lower transplant-free survival rates.[20] This correlation persisted regardless of underlying MELD score and HE grade in this particular study, but overall transplant-free survival was shown to be worse among patients with a MELD score above 15 or with a higher HE grade (**Fig. 3**). A randomized-controlled study from 2007 that examined the use of extracorporeal albumin dialysis in patients with HE and acute-on-chronic liver failure (ACLF) similarly demonstrated that the lack of improvement of HE within the first 5 days was associated with a worse survival in patients with a MELD score greater than 30.[21]

The presence of overt HE is also a prognostic indicator in patients with cirrhosis after placement of transjugular intrahepatic portosystemic shunt (TIPS). Based on retrospective data published in 2019, early recurrence of overt HE (defined as HE occurring within 3 months) was associated with an increased risk of mortality in patients after TIPS even after adjustment for age, MELD score, presence of ascites, and TIPS indication. When early overt HE was further divided into early recurrent HE and a single episode of HE, death was more common in patients with early recurrent episodes of HE over the course of the study period.[22]

The presence of overt HE in hospitalized patients with cirrhosis also has prognostic significance. Overall mortality has been shown to be higher in hospitalized patients with cirrhosis and HE, and the association between the presence of HE and higher mortality is independent of other organ failures.[23] Higher mortality rates were also seen at 28, 90, and 365 days after hospitalization in patients with decompensated

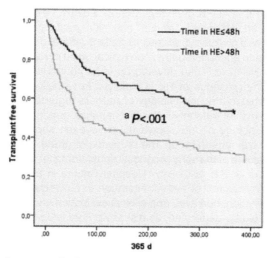

Fig. 3. Transplant-free survival of patients included in the study in relation to time in HE. Patients with a time in HE >48h versus those with time in HE≤48h presented lower transplant-free survival rates at any time point with [a] P<.001 at 28, 90 and 365 days. HE, hepatic encephalopathy. (*From* Ventura-Cots M, Carmona I, Moreno C, et al. Duration of the acute hepatic encephalopathy episode determines survival in cirrhotic patients. Ther Adv Gastroenterol 2018; 11: 1-12; with permission.)

cirrhosis and HE compared to those without HE (**Fig. 4**).[24] The association between HE and higher mortality in hospitalized patients is particularly strong in ACLF, and multiple prospective and retrospective studies have demonstrated this association.[25] The degree of mental impairment additionally has prognostic implications, and more severe encephalopathy portends a higher mortality risk in ACLF.[26] This is similar to patients who develop acute liver failure (ALF) in that worse HE grade not only correlates with but defines a worsening clinical status.

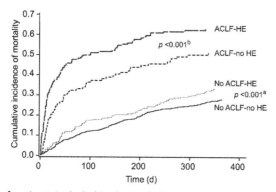

Fig. 4. Mortality of patients included in the study in relation to the presence of HE or ACLF (alone or in combination) at inclusion (competitive risk assessment). [a] P value comparing presence versus absence of hepatic encephalopathy in patients without ACLF; [b] P value comparing presence versus absence of hepatic encephalopathy in patients with ACLF. (*From* Cordoba J, Ventura-Cots M, Simon-Talero M, et al. Characteristics, risk factors, and mortality of cirrhotic patients hospitalized for hepatic encephalopathy with and without acute-on-chronic liver failure. J Hepatol 2014; 60: 275-281; with permission.)

The presence of HE in ALF is often regarded as a distinct entity from HE in decompensated cirrhosis, and HE in ALF arguably has even greater prognostic value. ALF is commonly defined as a clinical syndrome in a patient without pre-existing liver disease with coagulopathy and encephalopathy. The typical onset of HE in patients with ALF is 1 to 2 weeks, but HE in ALF can develop up to 6 months later and still meet ALF criteria. Although the presence of HE is included in virtually all definitions of ALF, the grade of encephalopathy and etiology of ALF are regarded as the 2 key factors that determine the overall outcome.[27] Higher hepatic coma grades (grade 3 and 4), regardless of the etiology of ALF, however, have been shown to result in worse transplant-free survival rates (**Fig. 5**). The presence of grade 3 or 4 encephalopathy was also found to be one of the early prognostic indicators that is potentially more useful than MELD score or King's College Hospital Criteria in predicting adverse outcomes in ALF.[28] Any degree of mental alteration in suspected ALF should prompt immediate hospitalization, however, and clinical evaluation and consideration for liver transplantation should be performed, as disease progression is often rapid once any disturbance in cognition is present.[29]

RISK FACTORS FOR POOR PROGNOSIS IN HEPATIC ENCEPHALOPATHY

Multiple studies have been able to identify particular risk factors associated with poor prognosis in patients with HE. A prospective study of hospitalized patients with HE demonstrated that patients with hyponatremia and acid-base disturbances tended to have a poor prognosis compared with the control group.[30] This increased mortality was specifically associated with patients who presented with a pH of less than 7.3 or greater than 7.55. Prior retrospective data from cirrhotic patients who developed an initial episode of HE have also demonstrated that male gender, worse renal function,

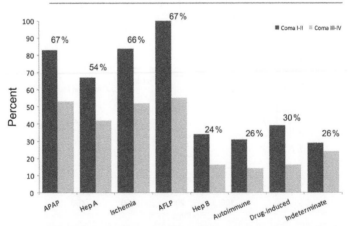

Fig. 5. Outcomes according to etiology and coma grade. The bars for each etiology indicate the percent survival without transplantation according to coma grade (I,II vs III,IV). The percent above each pair indicates the overall percentage of spontaneous survival for that etiology. There is a disparity between the etiologies with good survival and those with poor survival, but survival is much poorer in all categories if the patient is admitted with an advanced coma grade. (*From* Lee WM. Recent developments in acute liver failure. Best Pract Res Clin Gastroenterol 2012; 26: 3-16; with permission.)

increased serum bilirubin, decreased prothrombin activity, increased potassium, and decreased serum albumin were independently associated with a poor prognosis.[18] Many similar factors correlated with a worse prognosis in patients with ACLF and HE in a retrospective study, and these factors included higher stage of HE, presence of hepatorenal syndrome, and reduced prothrombin activity.[31]

There are also data to suggest that the presence of HE plays a greater prognostic role in ACLF patients than in patients with decompensated cirrhosis.[24] In a retrospective study of hospitalized patients with acute decompensation, prognosis was relatively preserved in patients with acute decompensated cirrhosis who developed HE. Patients with ACLF who developed HE were found to have an extremely poor prognosis, however, and independent risk factors of mortality in this group were similar to those found in other studies and included age, bilirubin, international normalized ratio (INR), creatinine, sodium, and HE grade.

POST-TRANSPLANT OUTCOMES IN PATIENTS WITH HEPATIC ENCEPHALOPATHY

Post-transplant encephalopathy is a relatively frequent complication that can be caused by a variety of etiologies including allograft dysfunction, medication toxicity, infection, metabolic derangements, and cerebrovascular events.[32] Retrospective data have demonstrated a higher risk of post-transplant encephalopathy in patients with a history of severe HE in the pre-transplant setting. The presence of active preoperative HE was also the strongest predictor of postoperative morbidity. This suggests that the presence of overt HE in pre-transplant patients can serve as a prognostic marker, not only for pre-transplant outcomes, but also for post-transplant outcomes.[33]

The presence of HE in the pre-transplant period also seems to impact neurocognitive function in the post-transplant period, even if post-transplant encephalopathy is not present. In a cohort study of patients with cirrhosis who underwent orthotopic liver transplantation (OLT), patients with overt HE in the pre-transplant period seemed to suffer more overall neurocognitive abnormalities in the post-transplant period compared to those without overt HE prior to transplant.[34] These differences occurred based on psychometric testing performed at an average of 18 months after OLT (**Fig. 6**), but the neurocognitive abnormalities did not appear to impact quality of life

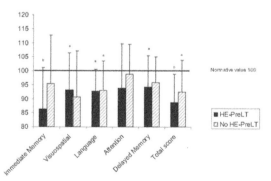

Fig. 6. Repeatable Battery for the Assessment of Neuropsychological Status (RBANS) results of both groups of patients compared with normative values. [a] $P<.05$, [b] $P<.001$. (*From* Sotil EU, Gottstein J, Ayala E, et al. Impact of preoperative overt hepatic encephalopathy on neurocognitive function after liver transplantation. Liver Transpl 2009; 15: 184-192; with permission.)

in this particular study. A prospective study of patients with cirrhosis who underwent liver transplant similarly identified an abnormal neurologic examination before transplant to be an independent risk factor for developing in-hospital central nervous system complications after transplant.[35] Additional prospective data published in 2010 corroborated this finding and demonstrated that pre-transplant HE had an effect on cognitive function after OLT, and this was thought to be at least in part due to associated brain volume and neuronal loss.[36] Cross-sectional data have also supported the notion that episodes of HE may have persistent and cumulative deficits that are chronic and not readily reversible after liver transplantation.[37]

Even the presence of subclinical HE in the pre-transplant period may have neurologic implications on post-transplant outcomes. Limited prospective data demonstrate persistent cognitive dysfunction and radiologic abnormalities in post-transplant patients with minimal HE before OLT.[38] A longitudinal study of patients with subclinical HE in 2004 also demonstrated the persistence of multiple neurocognitive deficits after transplant, and many specific cognitive functions such as verbal short-term memory required up to 18 months to improve after OLT was performed.[39]

Improvement of Outcomes After Therapy of Hepatic Encephalopathy

Treatment of HE with conventional therapies including rifaximin and lactulose has been associated with improved clinical outcomes. Rifaximin therapy in conjunction with lactulose use has been shown to significantly reduce the risk of an episode of HE over a 6-month period, and the addition of rifaximin was also shown to significantly reduce the risk of hospitalization because of HE by nearly 10% compared with the placebo group.[40] Subsequent data have also demonstrated lower hospitalization rates with rifaximin use and decreased duration of hospitalization, lower hospital costs, and fewer associated adverse events.[41] Treatment of overt HE with rifaximin and lactulose has also been associated with a nearly 20% decrease in mortality in the pre-transplant setting compared to treatment with lactulose alone.[42]

Therapy of HE in the pre-transplant setting may be used for subclinical HE, overt HE, and the prevention of HE relapse given the association of subclinical and overt HE to worsened clinical outcomes and increased mortality, but treatment of subclinical HE is not currently routine outside the context of clinical trials.[43] Underlying cognitive impairment may still persist despite resolution of overt HE on therapy,[37] however, and the full significance of these residual neurocognitive deficits in the pre-transplant and post-transplant settings has yet to be fully elucidated.

SUMMARY

The development of HE is an important prognostic indicator for clinical outcomes in decompensated cirrhosis, ALF, and liver transplant recipients. Overt HE has long been acknowledged as a prognostic marker associated with increased hospitalizations and worse survival, but recent data have also highlighted the clinical importance of diagnosing subclinical HE by psychometric testing. Patients with subclinical HE are more likely to develop overt HE, and these patients have a similarly higher risk of falls, motor vehicle accidents, hospitalizations, and mortality compared to cirrhotic patients without subclinical HE. Even a single episode of HE portends shorter life expectancies, and the development of HE has worse 1-year mortality rates compared with other markers of hepatic decompensation. The duration of an episode of HE and the grade of HE impact overall survival in decompensated cirrhosis, and the higher grade of HE is also associated with worse transplant-free survival rates in ALF.

There are several risk factors for poor prognosis associated in HE, and these variables in prior publications have included male gender, older age, higher bilirubin, worse renal function, and reduced prothrombin activity. The presence of severe HE in the perioperative setting also tends to be associated with the presence of encephalopathy after liver transplantation, and the presence of active HE prior to liver transplantation is a strong predictor for postoperative mortality based on retrospective data. The presence of subclinical HE may also have neurologic impacts after liver transplantation, but the clinical significance of this has yet to be fully elucidated. Conventional therapy of overt HE with rifaximin and lactulose has been shown to reduce the recurrence of HE, as well as associated hospitalizations and mortality, but treatment of subclinical HE is not nearly as routinely prescribed despite the increasing body of literature demonstrating its similar clinical burden.

DISCLOSURE

The authors have nothing to disclose.

REFERENCES

1. Bajaj JS. Minimal hepatic encephalopathy matters in daily life. World J Gastroenterol 2008;14:23.
2. Prasad S, Dhiman RK, Duseja A, et al. Lactulose improves cognitive functions and health-related quality of life in patients with cirrhosis who have minimal hepatic encephalopathy. Hepatology 2007;45:549–59.
3. Meyer T, Eshelman A, Abouljoud M. Neuropsychological changes in a large sample of liver transplant candidates. Transplant Proc 2006;38:3559–60.
4. Groeneweg M, Quero JC, De Brujin I, et al. Subclinical hepatic encephalopathy impairs daily functioning. Hepatology 1998;28:45–9.
5. Stewart CA, Smith GE. Minimal hepatic encephalopathy. Nat Clin Pract Gastroenterol Hepatol 2007;4:677–85.
6. Roman E, Cordoba J, Torrens M, et al. Minimal hepatic encephalopathy is associated with falls. Am J Gastroenterol 2011;106:476–82.
7. Bajaj JS, Saeian K, Schubert CM, et al. Minimal hepatic encephalopathy is associated with motor vehicle crashes: the reality beyond the driving test. Hepatol 2010;50:1175–83.
8. Wein C, Koch H, Popp B, et al. Minimal hepatic encephalopathy impairs fitness to drive. Hepatol 2004;39:739–45.
9. Patidar KR, Thacker LR, Wade JB, et al. Covert hepatic encephalopathy is independently associated with poor survival and increased risk of hospitalization. Am J Gastroenterol 2014;109:1757–63.
10. Romero-Gomez M, Boza F, Garcia-Valdecasas MS, et al. Subclinical hepatic encephalopathy predicts the development of over hepatic encephalopathy. Am J Gastroenterol 2001;96:2718–23.
11. Yen CL. Somatosensory evoked potentials and number connection test in detection of subclinical hepatic encephalopathy. Hepatogastroenterology 1990;37:332–4.
12. Das A, Dhiman RK, Saraswat VA, et al. Prevalence and natural history of subclinical hepatic encephalopathy in cirrhosis. J Gastroenterol Hepatol 2001;16:531–5.
13. Romero-Gomez M, Grande L, Camacho I, et al. Altered response to oral glutamine challenge as prognostic factor for overt episodes in patients with minimal hepatic encephalopathy. Liver 2002;22:190–7.

14. Hartmann IJ, Groeneweg M, Quero JC, et al. The prognostic significance of subclinical hepatic encephalopathy. Am J Gastroenterol 2000;95:2029–34.
15. Dhiman RK, Kurmi R, Thumburu KK, et al. Diagnosis and prognostic significance of minimal hepatic encephalopathy in patients with cirrhosis of liver. Dig Dis Sci 2010;55:2381–90.
16. Child CG, Turcotte JG. Surgery and portal hypertension. Major Probl Clin Surg 1964;1:1–85.
17. Pugh RN, Murray-Lyon IM, Dawson JL, et al. Transection of the esophagus for bleeding oesophageal varices. Br J Surg 1973;60:646–9.
18. Bustamante J, Rimola A, Ventura PJ, et al. Prognostic significance of hepatic encephalopathy in patients with cirrhosis. J Hepatol 1999;30:890–5.
19. Jepsen P, Ott P, Andersen PK, et al. Clinical course of alcoholic liver cirrhosis: a Danish population-based cohort study. Hepatol 2010;51:1675–82.
20. Ventura-Cots M, Carmona I, Moreno C, et al. Duration of the acute hepatic encephalopathy episode determines survival in cirrhotic patients. Therap Adv Gastroenterol 2018;11:1–12.
21. Hassanein TI, Tofteng F, Brown RS Jr, et al. Randomized controlled study of extracorporeal albumin dialysis for hepatic encephalopathy in advanced cirrhosis. Hepatol 2007;46:1853–62.
22. Zuo L, Iv Y, Wang Q, et al. Early-recurrent overt hepatic encephalopathy is associated with reduced survival in cirrhotic patients after transjugular intrahepatic portosystemic shunt creation. J Vasc Interv Radiol 2019;30:148–53.
23. Romero-Gomez M, Montagnese S, Jalan R. Hepatic encephalopathy in patients with acute decompensation of cirrhosis and acute-on-chronic liver failure. J Hepatol 2015;62:437–47.
24. Cordoba J, Ventura-Cots M, Simon-Talero M, et al. Characteristics, risk factors, and mortality of cirrhotic patients hospitalized for hepatic encephalopathy with and without acute-on-chronic liver failure. J Hepatol 2014;60:275–81.
25. Lee GH. Hepatic encephalopathy in acute-on-chronic liver failure. Hepatolol Int 2015;9:520.
26. Amodio P. Hepatic encephalopathy: diagnosis and management. Liver Int 2018; 38:966–75.
27. Lee WM. Recent developments in acute liver failure. Best Pract Res Clin Gastroenterol 2012;26:3–16.
28. Dhiman RK, Jain S, Maheshwari U, et al. Early indicators of prognosis in fulminant hepatic failure: an assessment of the model for end-stage liver disease (MELD) and King's College Hospital Criteria. Liver Transpl 2006;13:814–21.
29. Lee WM, Schiødt FV. Fulminant hepatic failure. In: Schiff ER, Sorrell MF, Maddrey WC, editors. Schiff's diseases of the liver. 8th edition. Philadelphia: Lippincott-Raven Publishers; 1999. p. 879–95.
30. Chengshan R, Lei W, Xiaoyan Z, et al. Hepatic encephalopathy complicated with hyponatremia and acid-base disturbance and its prognosis. Journal of Medical Colleges of PLA 2012;27:143–60.
31. Yanping CUI. Logistic regression analysis of prognostic factors in 106 acute-on-chronic liver failure patients with hepatic encephalopathy. Lin Chuang Gan Dan Bing Za Zhi 2014;30:992–5.
32. Wijdicks EF. Impaired consciousness after liver transplantation. Liver Transpl Surg 1995;1:329–34.
33. Dhar R, Young GB, Marotta P. Perioperative neurological complications after liver transplantation are best predicted by pre-transplant hepatic encephalopathy. Neurocrit Care 2008;8:253–8.

34. Sotil EU, Gottstein J, Ayala E, et al. Impact of preoperative overt hepatic encephalopathy on neurocognitive function after liver transplantation. Liver Transpl 2009; 15:184–92.
35. Pujol A, Graus F, Rimola A, et al. Predictive factors of in-hospital CNS complications following liver transplantation. Neurology 1994;44:1226–30.
36. Garcia-Martinez R, Rovira A, Alonso J, et al. Hepatic encephalopathy is associated with posttransplant cognitive function and brain volume. Liver Transpl 2010;17:38–46.
37. Bajaj JS, Schubert CM, Heuman DM, et al. Persistence of cognitive impairment after resolution of overt hepatic encephalopathy. Gastroenterology 2010;138: 2332–40.
38. Mechtcheriakov S, Graziadei IW, Mattedi M, et al. Incomplete improvement of visuo-motor deficits in patients with minimal hepatic encephalopathy after liver transplantation. Liver Transpl 2004;10:77–83.
39. Mattarozzi K, Stracciari A, Vignatelli R, et al. Minimal hepatic encephalopathy: longitudinal effects of liver transplantation. Arch Neurol 2004;61:242–7.
40. Bass NM, Mullen KD, Sanyal A, et al. Rifaximin treatment in hepatic encephalopathy. N Engl J Med 2010;362:1071–81.
41. Leevy CB, Phillips JA. Hospitalizations during the use of rifaximin versus lactulose for the treatment of hepatic encephalopathy. Dig Dis Sci 2007;52:737–41.
42. Sharma BC, Sharma P, Lunia MK, et al. A randomized, double-blind, controlled trial comparing rifaximin plus lactulose with lactulose alone in treatment of overt hepatic encephalopathy. Am J Gastroenterol 2013;108:1458–63.
43. Teperman LW. Impact of pretransplant hepatic encephalopathy on liver post-transplantation outcomes. Int J Hepatol 2013;2013:1–9.

Pharmacologic Management of Hepatic Encephalopathy

Noah Y. Mahpour, MD[a], Lauren Pioppo-Phelan, MD[a], Mishal Reja, MD[a], Augustine Tawadros, MD[a], Vinod K. Rustgi, MD, MBA[b],*

KEYWORDS

- Lactulose • FMT • L-ornithine L-aspartate • Branched chain amino acid
- Ornithine phenylacetate • L-carnitine • Zinc • Acarbose

KEY POINTS

- Laxatives, such as lactulose, and antibiotics, such as rifaximin, have strong evidence behind them, and are associated with reduced severity, length, and frequency of encephalopathy.
- New research and therapeutics exist, including fecal transplants.
- New research and therapeutics exist also include small molecule therapies, such as branched chain amino acids.

INTRODUCTION

Pharmacologic management of hepatic encephalopathy includes a broad array of therapies, both established and experimental. Although there are specific mainstays, such as antibiotics and laxatives, with an established evidence base, there are newer, more radical modalities, such as bioartificial support systems, which could well become the next wave of hepatic support systems with significant reduction in encephalopathy secondary to the liver. In this article, we review current and potentially new pharmacologic therapies used in the management of hepatic encephalopathy.

LAXATIVES

Laxatives are widely used in the treatment of hepatic encephalopathy. Lactulose and lactitol are the most commonly used synthetic disaccharides. The available data suggest that approximately 70% to 80% of patients with hepatic encephalopathy improve with lactulose treatment.[1–3] Lactulose is widely available, but lactitol is not available in some countries (including the United States). Treatment with lactulose or lactitol is

[a] Department of Internal Medicine, Robert Wood Johnson School of Medicine, 1 Robert Wood Johnson Place, New Brunswick, NJ 08901, USA; [b] Center for Liver Diseases and Liver Masses, Robert Wood Johnson School of Medicine, MedEd Building, Room 466, 1 Robert Wood Johnson Place, New Brunswick, NJ 08901, USA
* Corresponding author.
E-mail address: vr262@rwjms.rutgers.edu

Clin Liver Dis 24 (2020) 231–242
https://doi.org/10.1016/j.cld.2020.01.005
1089-3261/20/© 2020 Elsevier Inc. All rights reserved.

based on the absence of a specific disaccharidase on the microvillus membrane of enterocytes in the human small bowel, thereby permitting entry of the disaccharides into the colon. Bacteria in the colon catabolize lactulose (beta-galactosidofructose) and lactitol (beta-galactosidosorbitol) to short chain fatty acids (eg, lactic acid and acetic acid), lowering the colonic pH to approximately 5. The reduction in pH favors the formation of the nonabsorbable ammonium from ammonia, trapping ammonium in the colon and thus decreasing plasma ammonia concentrations. Additionally, these laxatives increase the incorporation of ammonia by bacteria for synthesis of nitrogenous compounds, modify the colonic flora, and displase urease-producing bacteria with non–urease-producing Lactobacillus.[4] The cathartic effects of a hyperosmolar load in the colon improves gastrointestinal transit, allowing less time for ammonia absorption, with increased fecal nitrogen excretion ($\leq$4-fold) with an increase in stool volume.[5] Finally, the decreased formation of potentially toxic short chain fatty acids (eg, propionate, butyrate, valerate) is theorized to aid in encephalopathy symptoms.[6]

The dose of medication should be titrated to achieve 2 to 3 soft stools per day. Typically, lactulose is given as 30 to 45 mL (20–30 g) 2 to 4 times per day. An equivalent dose of lactitol is approximately 67 to 100 g of powder diluted in 100 mL of water. Treatment is usually well-tolerated, with principal side effects including abdominal cramping, diarrhea, and flatulence. Lactulose and lactitol may also be given as enemas in patients who are unable to take them orally (1–3 L of a 20% solution). The average price of 473 mL 10 g/15 mL of lactulose oral solution is $34.23.

A systematic review found that the use of lactulose or lactitol was more effective than placebo in improving hepatic encephalopathy (relative risk of no improvement, 0.6; 95% confidence interval, 0.5–0.8), but did not improve survival.[7]

Lactulose has also been studied for the prevention of recurrent hepatic encephalopathy. In a randomized trial with 140 patients who had recovered from hepatic encephalopathy, patients assigned to lactulose (30–60 mL in 2–3 divided doses titrated to 2–3 soft stools per day) had significantly fewer episodes of recurrent overt hepatic encephalopathy than patients who received placebo during 14 months of follow-up (20% vs 47%).[8] However, there were no significant differences in deaths or rates of readmission for causes other than hepatic encephalopathy.

Disaccharide enemas are also effective for removing ammoniagenic substrates from the colon. A randomized trial of 20 patients with hepatic encephalopathy suggested that 1 to 3 L of a 20% lactose or lactitol solution given as an enema was more effective than tap water enemas.[9] A possible explanation for this finding is that colonic acidification rather than bowel cleansing was the therapeutic mechanism.

It is unclear whether the route of administration of nonabsorbable disaccharides alters their efficacy. However, the convenience of oral administration generally makes it the preferred route.

Most trials of disaccharides included patients with overt hepatic encephalopathy. However, the use of nonabsorbable disaccharides may also benefit patients with minimal hepatic encephalopathy.[10,11] One trial that showed this included 61 patients with minimal hepatic encephalopathy.[12] Treatment with lactulose was associated with improvement in health-related quality of life and cognitive function. However, other trials have failed to show a benefit of treating patients with minimal hepatic encephalopathy. As a result, whether treatment should be routine in patients with minimal hepatic encephalopathy is unclear.

Polyethylene glycol (PEG) solution is a cathartic that may help to treat hepatic encephalopathy by increasing excretion of ammonia in the stool. PEG was compared with lactulose in a trial that included patients with cirrhosis who were admitted to the hospital with hepatic encephalopathy.[13] Patients were randomly assigned to receive 4 L of PEG over 4 hours or lactulose (≥3 doses of 20–30 g over 24 hours). After 24 hours, patients who received PEG had more improvement in their hepatic encephalopathy scoring algorithm score compared with those who received lactulose (from a mean score of 2.3 to 0.9 compared with 2.3 to 1.6). In addition, the median time to resolution of the hepatic encephalopathy was shorter with PEG (1 vs 2 days). The average price of a standard solution of PEG (3350 powder solution 527 g) is $37.74.

FECAL MICROBIOTA TRANSPLANT

Fecal microbiota transplant (FMT) is a commonly used treatment of overt hepatic encephalopathy refractory to standard medical management. It is well-proven that the ammonia generated by enteric bacteria is a critical driver of hepatic encephalopathy. The microbiota in patients with liver cirrhosis have more urease-producing bacteria, associated with increased production of ammonia and lipopolysaccharide. Therefore, by manipulating the gut microbiome through FMT, there is potential to reverse intestinal dysbiosis, resulting in cognitive improvement in overt hepatic encephalopathy.

Two trials that studied the efficacy of FMT in hepatic encephalopathy demonstrated that FMT improved outcomes. In 1 trial, 20 patients were randomized in a 1:1 ratio to standard of care (SOC) alone or SOC plus 5 days of pretreatment with broad-spectrum antibiotics followed by a single FMT enema from a single donor. The primary end point was safety based on FMT-related serious adverse events. A secondary end point was improvement in cognition. At baseline, both groups were similar in terms of demographics, past hepatic encephalopathy history, and liver function. The FMT group had a significantly lower rate of serious adverse events compared with the SOC-only group (20% vs 80%), and none were FMT related. Furthermore, during the follow-up period, none of the FMT patients developed hepatic encephalopathy, compared with 5 (50%) in the SOC-only group (P = .03). There was improvement in cognition from baseline in the FMT group, but not the SOC-only group.[14]

The second trial was an open-label, randomized clinical trial with a 5-month follow-up in outpatient men with cirrhosis with recurrent hepatic encephalopathy on SOC.[15] FMT randomized patients received 5 days of broad-spectrum antibiotic pretreatment, then a single FMT enema from the same donor with the optimal microbiota deficient in hepatic encephalopathy. Follow-up occurred on days 5, 6, 12, 35, and 150 after randomization. The primary outcome was safety of FMT compared with SOC using FMT-related serious adverse events. Secondary outcomes were adverse events, cognition, microbiota, and metabolic changes. Participants in both arms were similar on all baseline criteria and were followed until study end. FMT with antibiotic pretreatment was well-tolerated. Eight SOC participants (80%) had a total of 11 serious adverse events compared with 2 FMT participants (20%) with serious adverse events (both FMT unrelated; P = .02). Five SOC and no FMT participants developed further hepatic encephalopathy (P = .03). Cognition improved in the FMT, but not the SOC, group. The Model for End-Stage Liver Disease score worsened transiently after antibiotics, but reverted to baseline after FMT.

FMT is a safe and efficient treatment for hepatic encephalopathy. One of the main deterrents of FMT is its average cost of $1223. After failed medical management, the cost is more likely to become a secondary issue.

L-ORNITHINE L-ASPARTATE

L-Ornithine L-aspartate (LOLA) is the stable salt of amino acids ornithine and aspartate, and has been found to be effective in hepatic encephalopathy. It works via a substrate mechanism on the liver and skeletal muscle. Carbamoyl phosphate synthetase and glutamine synthetase are both key enzymes for urea and glutamine synthesis, respectively. In a cirrhosis state, these enzymes are impaired, resulting in hyperammonemia. Ornithine activates carbamoyl phosphate synthetase in the liver, and both ornithine and aspartate act peripherally by stimulating glutamine synthesis via glutamine synthetase.[16,17] A 2018 Cochrane meta-analysis of 29 trials involving 1891 participants examined LOLA compared with placebo and other anti–hepatic encephalopathy treatments. It was found that LOLA demonstrated improvement in mortality (relative risk [RR], 0.42), hepatic encephalopathy (RR, 0.7), and prevention of serious adverse effects (RR, 0.63) when compared with placebo or no treatment. However, it also found no benefit when compared with other anti–hepatic encephalopathy treatments, including lactulose, rifaximin, probiotics, or branched chain amino acids (BCAAs). In subgroup analysis, pooled data from 9 trials showed significant reduction in venous ammonia with either intravenous or oral LOLA. Oral LOLA was shown to be superior for minimal hepatic encephalopathy. The dose and duration is varied across studies and routes of administration. Oral dosages have ranged between 9 and 18 g/d in previous trials, and intravenous dosages between 20 and 30 g/d for 3 to 8 days. Overall, the quality of evidence was low, and additional data and further investigation are needed.[18]

A 2017 randomized, controlled trial found intravenous LOLA to be effective in reverting overt hepatic encephalopathy at day 5 of treatment when compared with placebo, as well as decreasing the duration of hospitalization and length of treatment.[19] A separate randomized, controlled trial of 63 cirrhotic patients showed LOLA 5 g 3 times per day for 60 days did not treat cognitive deficits, but did prevent future overt hepatic encephalopathy episodes at 6 months.[20]

To date, no trials have assessed the cost effectiveness of LOLA, but ongoing trials are continuing to study recovery and hospital stay. LOLA is available in oral supplement form over the counter. Intravenous LOLA (Hepa-merz) is available in Europe and other countries outside of the United States. It must be obtained with a prescription at a pharmacy and can be administered at an infusion center.

BRANCHED CHAIN AMINO ACIDS

The BCAAs (isoleucine, leucine, and valine) have attracted particular attention for their therapeutic efficacy in hepatic encephalopathy. The pathophysiology of these molecules in hepatic encephalopathy is not yet fully understood. Previously, it had been suggested that decreased BCAAs resulted in an increase ratio of aromatic amino acids to BCAA. This led to an increased number of aromatic amino acids crossing the blood–brain barrier, leading to inefficient dopaminergic neurotransmission.[21] However, it is now believed that BCAAs aid in detoxification of ammonia by its effects on skeletal muscle. Skeletal muscle detoxifies ammonia via conversion to glutamine. In cirrhosis, hyperammonemia impairs skeletal muscle protein synthesis via alteration of mTOR signaling; BCAAs have been shown to counteract this pathway.[22]

A 2016 Cochrane review examined the effects of BCAAs on hepatic encephalopathy. Sixteen randomized, controlled trials including 827 participants classified as having overt hepatic encephalopathy (12 trials) or minimal hepatic encephalopathy (4 trials). Eight trials assessed BCAA supplements and 7 trials assessed intravenous BCAA. It found that BCAAs had a beneficial effect on manifestations of hepatic encephalopathy, with a number needed to treat of 5 patients and an RR of 0.73. No significant effect was found on mortality, quality of life, or nutritional measures.[23]

ORNITHINE PHENYLACETATE

Ornithine phenylacetate works to decrease ammonia by focusing on the production of glutamate and the removal of glutamine. L-ornithine stimulates glutamine synthetase peripherally to produce glutamine. The glutamine is then conjugated by phenylacetate to form phenylacetylglutamine, which is then excreted by the urine.[24,25] One randomized, controlled trial of 38 cirrhotic patients enrolled within 24 hours of an upper gastrointestinal bleed indicated that ornithine phenylacetate did not significantly decrease plasma ammonia.[26]

L-CARNITINE

Carnitine has been shown to be protective against ammonia neurotoxicity.[27] It is a metabolite of lysine, and carries short chain fatty acids across the mitochondrial membrane. In an randomized, controlled trial of 67 patients with minimal hepatic encephalopathy, those who received L-carnitine had significantly improved energy level and well-being.[28] A randomized, controlled trial of 121 patients with overt hepatic encephalopathy showed significant improvement in markers of both mild and moderate hepatic encephalopathy.[20]

ZINC

Zinc has been thought to enhance neurotransmission and aid in hepatic conversion of amino acids into urea. Cirrhotic patients have been shown to be commonly zinc deficient.[29,30] In a randomized, controlled trial of 79 patients on polaprezinc (zinc + L-carnosine), 25 patients showed significant improvement in hepatic encephalopathy as compared with standard therapies. Oral zinc alone was not found to decrease hepatic encephalopathy recurrence.[31,32]

DOPAMINERGIC AGENTS

Patients with hepatic encephalopathy frequently complain of extrapyramidal symptoms, and have been shown to have alterations in their basal ganglia. A Cochrane analysis in 2014 examined 3 trials with levodopa and 2 trials with bromocriptine in 144 patients with hepatic encephalopathy. No significant differences were found in symptoms or mortality.[33]

OTHER NEUROTRANSMITTERS

Two experimental rat models have shown NMDA overactivity in hepatic encephalopathy. Memantine, an NMDA antagonist, showed significant improvement in clinical grading of hepatic encephalopathy and less slowing on an electroencephalogram, but no change in ammonia levels.[34] Serotonin has been shown to increase cerebral concentrations in hepatic encephalopathy, and 5HT1A and 5HT2 receptors are altered.[35,36] Nonselective serotonin receptor antagonist methysergine increase motor activity in stages 2 to 3 hepatic encephalopathy.[37]

ACARBOSE

Acarbose is a competitive inhibitor of the alpha-amylase (pancreatic enzyme) and alpha-glucoside (intestinal enzyme). By reducing the digestion of complex starches to their smaller mono and disaccharide components, acarbose lowers blood glucose concentrations in patients with type 2 diabetes mellitus secondary to the intestine's inability to absorb the molecules. As a proposed mechanism of action in hepatic encephalopathy, acarbose is hypothesized to improve mentation through a secondary effect, because the improvements in glucose levels are noted to improve cognitive functioning in patients. Additionally, it is theorized to decrease levels of intestinal bacteria flora that produce ammonia, among other active substances that may contribute to cognitive impairment.[38]

In 1 study investigating the effect of acarbose on improvement of hepatic encephalopathy (n = 107), there was a significant improvement in cognitive functioning, shown chiefly by improvement in the Reitan's Number Connection test.[38] In this limited study, including only patients with low-grade hepatic encephalopathy (grades 1–2), by using an 8-week treatment period with acarbose versus placebo, and calculating an Encephalopathy Global Score, demonstrable improvements were recorded. However, there were multiple limitations to study, including errors in calculations and a lack of generalizability, because the study population is actually quite rare in clinical practice, and the side effect profile of acarbose, including bloating, flatulence, and loose stools.[38]

One further report looking at improved glucose levels in type 2 diabetes and cirrhosis (well-compensated) showed improved glucose control through the use of acarbose; however, there was no investigation into effects on hepatic encephalopathy. There is mention of a noted improvement of ammonia levels, which could correlate with clinical evidence of encephalopathy, but further research would need to be undertaken.[39]

Even with weak evidence at best, a significantly limiting factor in the usage of acarbose is that a rare side effect of the medication is fulminant hepatitis, as well as elevated transaminases and bilirubin, reported by multiple investigators.[40]

FLUMAZENIL

Flumazenil is a benzodiazepine receptor antagonist often used in the setting of acute benzodiazepine overdose, to reverse the sedating effects of those pharmaceuticals. It acts primarily at the gamma aminobutyric acid receptor site, by inhibiting the binding of benzodiazepine molecules, without affecting the pharmacokinetics of the medication itself. In patients with hepatic encephalopathy, there have been theories that endogenous gamma aminobutyric acid-like molecules play a role in the development of encephalopathy. As such, there have been dedicated research efforts geared toward the use of flumazenil as an attempt to reverse some of the neurocognitive impairment displayed in hepatic encephalopathy.[41]

A 2004 Cochrane review of 13 trials, 3 of which were ultimately excluded, comparing flumazenil/benzodiazepine receptor antagonists versus placebo did not show any improvement in survival or recovery; however, 8 trials encompassing 766 patients showed symptomatic improvement in encephalopathy, based on varying assessments of mental status, ranging from the Glasgow Coma Scale to the Number Connection Test.[42]

In the 2017 update to the same Cochrane review, the authors search revealed 14 trials, only 12 of which were able to integrated into the data analysis (n = 842), that demonstrated again there was no change in mortality when using flumazenil in hepatic encephalopathy, but improvement in encephalopathy; however, assessment of improvement varied significantly between trials, the evidence was of low quality, and there was high risk of bias in all but 1 trial.[41]

Thus, based on the current evidence, it seems that flumazenil has a small benefit symptomatically in acute episodes of encephalopathy, especially in situations of benzodiazepine intoxication/overdose; further data are needed regarding the risks and benefits in other settings and populations.

BIOARTIFICIAL SUPPORT SYSTEMS

For the liver, support systems are akin to dialysis for patients requiring renal replacement, and can be divided into 2 broad categories: artificial liver support and bioartificial liver support. Artificial liver support removes circulating toxins via filtration, whereas bioartificial liver support uses filtration as well as liver cells to theoretically improve the detoxification process. Thus, in the treatment of hepatic encephalopathy, the theory behind using these support systems is intuitive, via detoxification of substrates ordinarily metabolized by a functioning liver.[43]

A 2004 Cochrane review of 14 trials compared support systems (artificial or bioartificial) for patients with acute or acute on chronic liver failure. The main focus was investigating the ability to bridge to recovery or liver transplantation, using these systems. Within the subgroup analysis, 12 of the 14 trials (n = 483) compared a support system with SOC medical therapy, and revealed that the use of a support system increased the odds of improving encephalopathy, with an RR of 0.67 (95% confidence interval, 0.52–0.86) compared with standard medical therapy.[44]

GLYCEROL PHENYLBUTYRATE

Traditionally used for patients with urea cycle metabolism disorders, glycerol phenylbutyrate, has been shown to provide an effective means for an alternative excretion point for urea in patients who are otherwise unable to do so.

A triglyceride molecule, glycerol phenylbutyrate contains 3 phenylbutyrate molecules, which are ultimately converted to the active molecule phenylacetate. Phenylacetate then is acetylated in the liver and kidneys, forming phenylacetylglutamine, thus providing an alternative path for nitrogen waste excretion in patients who cannot synthesize urea secondary to a urea cycle disorder.[45]

Early studies showed that glycerol phenylbutyrate administered as sodium phenylbutyrate was well-tolerated, and safe to use in patients with cirrhosis. Twenty-four healthy adults received glycerol phenylbutyrate and sodium phenylbutyrate, whereas 8 healthy adults and 24 patients with cirrhosis received single and multiple-day dosing of glycerol phenylbutyrate. Results showed that patients with cirrhosis converted glycerol phenylbutyrate to phenylacetylglutamine in a similar fashion to the healthy patients.[45]

Thus, a pilot study investigating the feasibility of using glycerol phenylbutyrate to lower ammonia levels in patients with cirrhosis in events of hepatic encephalopathy was developed. With promising results, specifically a significant reduction in serum ammonia levels using 6 mL of glycerol phenylbutyrate as treatment in the 15 patients enrolled, glycerol phenylbutyrate was investigated further.[46]

A randomized control trial was devised (n = 178), comparing glycerol phenylbutyrate versus placebo, with questionable benefits. In patients not taking rifaximin at the beginning of the study, there was a 22% relative risk reduction, but only a 2% absolute risk reduction (no significant difference). Overall, there was possibly a small benefit in hospitalizations with fewer hepatic encephalopathy hospitalizations (13 vs 25; $P = .06$) in the glycerol phenylbutyrate group, but similar numbers of hospital days and adverse events.[47] The study did not account well for the baseline differences for prior or concurrent treatments (rifaximin, lactulose), because patients were allowed to alter their treatment regimen if or when an episode of encephalopathy reoccurred. Additionally, significant differences existed in the baseline characteristics of the 2 groups (gender, severity of liver disease).[47]

ANTIMICROBIALS

Antimicrobials are widely used in the treatment of hepatic encephalopathy. As a review, hepatic encephalopathy is thought to be the result of rising levels of ammonia, which is produced by gut flora. Antibiotics can target these culprit gut flora, thus leading to decreased ammonia levels and the potential treatment of hepatic encephalopathy. However, prolonged use of antibiotics is associated with adverse effects that make this class of medication less ideal. Rifaximin is a synthetic antibiotic commonly used for the treatment of hepatic encephalopathy that provides antibacterial coverage against gram-negative and gram-positive bacteria, both aerobic and anaerobic. This antibiotic is an ideal choice, because it has a minimal rate of systemic absorption, thus obviating many adverse effects of prolonged systemic antimicrobial treatment.[48]

Antibiotics such as neomycin, vancomycin, and metronidazole have historically been used for treatment of hepatic encephalopathy. However, rifaximin has become the most widely used antibiotic for this indication owing to its safety, efficacy, and tolerability.[2,49] Although neomycin decreases the intestinal production of ammonia from glutamine, its clinical use is limited by its tendency to cause ototoxicity and nephrotoxicity.[50] Similarly, the use of vancomycin is limited by nephrotoxicity and risk of bacterial resistance, and long-term use of metronidazole is associated with nephrotoxicity and neurotoxicity.[50,51]

Rifaximin remains the most widely used antibiotic in the management of hepatic encephalopathy. A double-blind, randomized, placebo-controlled trial published in 2010 involving 299 patients in remission from hepatic encephalopathy revealed that rifaximin was more effective than placebo in preventing recurrent hepatic encephalopathy and hospitalization.[52] Furthermore, studies of safety and tolerability of rifaximin have shown no increase in adverse events, infection with *Clostridium difficile*, or bacterial antibiotic resistance.[53] Current guidelines recommend lactulose as the initial first-line treatment for hepatic encephalopathy; however, there is evidence that monotherapy with rifaximin can be effective, and rifaximin has been demonstrated to be noninferior to lactulose alone.[54–56]

For patients with severe hepatic encephalopathy or recurrent hepatic encephalopathy on lactulose, combination therapy with lactulose and rifaximin should be considered.[50,57] The combination of lactulose and rifaximin seems to be more effective than either drug alone. A recent randomized, controlled trial comparing lactulose plus rifaximin to lactulose alone found that more patients had complete resolution of hepatic encephalopathy than those treated with lactulose alone. These patients also had decreased mortality and hospital length of stay when compared with those on monotherapy.[58] Another recent literature review found that the addition of rifaximin to lactulose therapy decrease the risk of recurrence of overt hepatic encephalopathy and encephalopathy-related hospitalizations, and this combination is well-tolerated.[59]

PROBIOTICS

As previously, the gut microbiome plays an important role in hepatic encephalopathy, because gut bacteria are involved in the production of ammonia. Thus, it has been theorized that the use of probiotics to alter gut flora may be beneficial in the management of hepatic encephalopathy. There have been randomized, controlled trials that have compared probiotics to placebo, no treatment, or lactulose, which have demonstrated some benefit.[60–62] For secondary prophylaxis, a randomized, controlled trial comparing lactulose, probiotics, or no therapy revealed that, although both lactulose and probiotics were significantly more effective than no therapy, there was no significant difference between the 2 agents.[63] A systematic review of 9 randomized, controlled trials also showed that probiotics were associated with improvement of minimal hepatic encephalopathy, prevention of overt hepatic encephalopathy, and was also associated with a reduction in severe adverse events.[64] However, most data available are of low quality and there has been no evidence of any improvement in mortality.[65]

SUMMARY

The use of laxatives, such as lactulose, and antibiotics, such as rifaximin, have strong evidence behind them, and are associated with reduced severity, length, and frequency of encephalopathy.[7,58] Many new avenues of research and therapeutics exist, with fecal transplants, as well as other small molecule therapies, such as BCAAs, soon playing a vital role in the alleviation and prevention of Hepatic Encephalopathy.

DISCLOSURE

Authors have nothing to disclose.

REFERENCES

1. Ferenci P, Herneth A, Steindl P. Newer approaches to therapy of hepatic encephalopathy. Semin Liver Dis 1996;16(3):329–38.
2. Conn HO, Leevy CM, Vlahcevic ZR, et al. Comparison of lactulose and neomycin in the treatment of chronic portal-systemic encephalopathy. A double blind controlled trial. Gastroenterology 1977;72(4 Pt 1):573–83.
3. Sharma P, Sharma BC. Disaccharides in the treatment of hepatic encephalopathy. Metab Brain Dis 2013;28(2):313–20.
4. Riggio O, et al. Effect of lactitol and lactulose administration on the fecal flora in cirrhotic patients. J Clin Gastroenterol 1990;12(4):433–6.
5. Mortensen PB. The effect of oral-administered lactulose on colonic nitrogen metabolism and excretion. Hepatology 1992;16(6):1350–6.
6. Mortensen PB, et al. The degradation of amino acids, proteins, and blood to short-chain fatty acids in colon is prevented by lactulose. Gastroenterology 1990;98(2):353–60.
7. Als-Nielsen B, Gluud LL, Gluud C. Nonabsorbable disaccharides for hepatic encephalopathy. Cochrane Database Syst Rev 2004;(2):CD003044.
8. Sharma BC, et al. Secondary prophylaxis of hepatic encephalopathy: an open-label randomized controlled trial of lactulose versus placebo. Gastroenterology 2009;137(3):885–91, 891.e1.
9. Uribe M, et al. Acidifying enemas (lactitol and lactose) vs. nonacidifying enemas (tap water) to treat acute portal-systemic encephalopathy: a double-blind, randomized clinical trial. Hepatology 1987;7(4):639–43.
10. Prasad S, et al. Lactulose improves cognitive functions and health-related quality of life in patients with cirrhosis who have minimal hepatic encephalopathy. Hepatology 2007;45(3):549–59.
11. Watanabe A, et al. Clinical efficacy of lactulose in cirrhotic patients with and without subclinical hepatic encephalopathy. Hepatology 1997;26(6):1410–4.
12. Dhiman RK, et al. Efficacy of lactulose in cirrhotic patients with subclinical hepatic encephalopathy. Dig Dis Sci 2000;45(8):1549–52.
13. Rahimi RS, et al. Lactulose vs polyethylene glycol 3350–electrolyte solution for treatment of overt hepatic encephalopathy: the HELP randomized clinical trial. JAMA Intern Med 2014;174(11):1727–33.

14. Bajaj JS. The role of microbiota in hepatic encephalopathy. Gut Microbes 2014; 5(3):397–403.
15. Kao D, et al. Fecal microbiota transplantation in the management of hepatic encephalopathy. Hepatology 2016;63(1):339–40.
16. Acharya C, Bajaj JS. Current management of hepatic encephalopathy. Am J Gastroenterol 2018;113(11):1600–12.
17. Kircheis G, et al. Therapeutic efficacy of L-ornithine-L-aspartate infusions in patients with cirrhosis and hepatic encephalopathy: results of a placebo-controlled, double-blind study. Hepatology 1997;25(6):1351–60.
18. Goh ET, et al. L-ornithine L-aspartate for prevention and treatment of hepatic encephalopathy in people with cirrhosis. Cochrane Database Syst Rev 2018;(5):CD012410.
19. Sidhu SS, et al. L-ornithine L-aspartate in bouts of overt hepatic encephalopathy. Hepatology 2018;67(2):700–10.
20. Alvares-da-Silva MR, et al. Oral l-ornithine-l-aspartate in minimal hepatic encephalopathy: a randomized, double-blind, placebo-controlled trial. Hepatol Res 2014;44(9):956–63.
21. Dam G, et al. The role of branched chain amino acids in the treatment of hepatic Encephalopathy. J Clin Exp Hepatol 2018;8(4):448–51.
22. Tsien C, et al. Metabolic and molecular responses to leucine-enriched branched chain amino acid supplementation in the skeletal muscle of alcoholic cirrhosis. Hepatology 2015;61(6):2018–29.
23. Gluud LL, et al. Branched-chain amino acids for people with hepatic encephalopathy. Cochrane Database Syst Rev 2017;(5):CD001939.
24. Ventura-Cots M, et al. Safety of ornithine phenylacetate in cirrhotic decompensated patients: an open-label, dose-escalating, single-cohort study. J Clin Gastroenterol 2013;47(10):881–7.
25. Jover-Cobos M, et al. Ornithine phenylacetate targets alterations in the expression and activity of glutamine synthase and glutaminase to reduce ammonia levels in bile duct ligated rats. J Hepatol 2014;60(3):545–53.
26. Ventura-Cots M, et al. Impact of ornithine phenylacetate (OCR-002) in lowering plasma ammonia after upper gastrointestinal bleeding in cirrhotic patients. Therap Adv Gastroenterol 2016;9(6):823–35.
27. Hearn TJ, et al. Effect of orally administered L-carnitine on blood ammonia and L-carnitine concentrations in portacaval-shunted rats. Hepatology 1989;10(5): 822–8.
28. Malaguarnera M, et al. Acetyl-L-carnitine reduces depression and improves quality of life in patients with minimal hepatic encephalopathy. Scand J Gastroenterol 2011;46(6):750–9.
29. Loomba V, et al. Serum zinc levels in hepatic encephalopathy. Indian J Gastroenterol 1995;14(2):51–3.
30. Marchesini G, et al. Zinc supplementation and amino acid-nitrogen metabolism in patients with advanced cirrhosis. Hepatology 1996;23(5):1084–92.
31. Takuma Y, et al. Clinical trial: oral zinc in hepatic encephalopathy. Aliment Pharmacol Ther 2010;32(9):1080–90.
32. Chavez-Tapia NC, et al. A systematic review and meta-analysis of the use of oral zinc in the treatment of hepatic encephalopathy. Nutr J 2013;12:74.
33. Junker AE, et al. Dopamine agents for hepatic encephalopathy. Cochrane Database Syst Rev 2014;(2):CD003047.

34. Vogels BA, et al. Memantine, a noncompetitive NMDA receptor antagonist improves hyperammonemia-induced encephalopathy and acute hepatic encephalopathy in rats. Hepatology 1997;25(4):820–7.

35. Jellinger K, et al. Brain monoamines in human hepatic encephalopathy. Acta Neuropathol 1978;43(1–2):63–8.

36. Rao VL, Butterworth RF. Alterations of [3H]8-OH-DPAT and [3H]ketanserin binding sites in autopsied brain tissue from cirrhotic patients with hepatic encephalopathy. Neurosci Lett 1994;182(1):69–72.

37. Yurdaydin C, et al. Modulation of hepatic encephalopathy in rats with thioacetamide-induced acute liver failure by serotonin antagonists. Eur J Gastroenterol Hepatol 1996;8(7):667–71.

38. Gentile S, et al. A randomized controlled trial of acarbose in hepatic encephalopathy. Clin Gastroenterol Hepatol 2005;3(2):184–91.

39. Gentile S, et al. Effect of treatment with acarbose and insulin in patients with non-insulin-dependent diabetes mellitus associated with non-alcoholic liver cirrhosis. Diabetes Obes Metab 2001;3(1):33–40.

40. Hsiao SH, et al. Hepatotoxicity associated with acarbose therapy. Ann Pharmacother 2006;40(1):151–4.

41. Goh ET, et al. Flumazenil versus placebo or no intervention for people with cirrhosis and hepatic encephalopathy. Cochrane Database Syst Rev 2017;(7):CD002798.

42. Als-Nielsen B, Gluud LL, Gluud C. Benzodiazepine receptor antagonists for hepatic encephalopathy. Cochrane Database Syst Rev 2004;(2):CD002798.

43. MacDonald AJ, Karvellas CJ. Emerging role of extracorporeal support in acute and acute-on-chronic liver failure: recent developments. Semin Respir Crit Care Med 2018;39(5):625–34.

44. Liu JP, et al. Artificial and bioartificial support systems for liver failure. Cochrane Database Syst Rev 2004;(1):CD003628.

45. McGuire BM, et al. Pharmacology and safety of glycerol phenylbutyrate in healthy adults and adults with cirrhosis. Hepatology 2010;51(6):2077–85.

46. Ghabril M, et al. Glycerol phenylbutyrate in patients with cirrhosis and episodic hepatic encephalopathy: a pilot study of safety and effect on venous ammonia concentration. Clin Pharmacol Drug Dev 2013;2(3):278–84.

47. Rockey DC, et al. Randomized, double-blind, controlled study of glycerol phenylbutyrate in hepatic encephalopathy. Hepatology 2014;59(3):1073–83.

48. Festi D, et al. Management of hepatic encephalopathy: focus on antibiotic therapy. Digestion 2006;73(Suppl 1):94–101.

49. Suraweera D, Sundaram V, Saab S. Evaluation and management of hepatic encephalopathy: current status and future directions. Gut Liver 2016;10(4):509–19.

50. Leise MD, et al. Management of hepatic encephalopathy in the hospital. Mayo Clin Proc 2014;89(2):241–53.

51. Morgan MH, Read AE, Speller DC. Treatment of hepatic encephalopathy with metronidazole. Gut 1982;23(1):1–7.

52. Bass NM, et al. Rifaximin treatment in hepatic encephalopathy. N Engl J Med 2010;362(12):1071–81.

53. Mullen KD, et al. Rifaximin is safe and well tolerated for long-term maintenance of remission from overt hepatic encephalopathy. Clin Gastroenterol Hepatol 2014;12(8):1390–7.e2.

54. Vilstrup H, et al. Hepatic encephalopathy in chronic liver disease: 2014 practice guideline by the American Association for the Study of Liver Diseases and the European Association for the Study of the Liver. Hepatology 2014;60(2):715–35.

55. Neff GW, et al. Durability of rifaximin response in hepatic encephalopathy. J Clin Gastroenterol 2012;46(2):168–71.
56. Jiang Q, et al. Rifaximin versus nonabsorbable disaccharides in the management of hepatic encephalopathy: a meta-analysis. Eur J Gastroenterol Hepatol 2008; 20(11):1064–70.
57. Mohammad RA, Regal RE, Alaniz C. Combination therapy for the treatment and prevention of hepatic encephalopathy. Ann Pharmacother 2012;46(11):1559–63.
58. Sharma BC, et al. A randomized, double-blind, controlled trial comparing rifaximin plus lactulose with lactulose alone in treatment of overt hepatic encephalopathy. Am J Gastroenterol 2013;108(9):1458–63.
59. Hudson M, Schuchmann M. Long-term management of hepatic encephalopathy with lactulose and/or rifaximin: a review of the evidence. Eur J Gastroenterol Hepatol 2019;31(4):434–50.
60. Shavakhi A, et al. Multistrain probiotic and lactulose in the treatment of minimal hepatic encephalopathy. J Res Med Sci 2014;19(8):703–8.
61. Dhiman RK, et al. Probiotic VSL#3 reduces liver disease severity and hospitalization in patients with cirrhosis: a randomized, controlled trial. Gastroenterology 2014;147(6):1327–37.e3.
62. Lunia MK, et al. Probiotics prevent hepatic encephalopathy in patients with cirrhosis: a randomized controlled trial. Clin Gastroenterol Hepatol 2014;12(6): 1003–8.e1.
63. Agrawal A, et al. Secondary prophylaxis of hepatic encephalopathy in cirrhosis: an open-label, randomized controlled trial of lactulose, probiotics, and no therapy. Am J Gastroenterol 2012;107(7):1043–50.
64. Zhao LN, et al. Probiotics can improve the clinical outcomes of hepatic encephalopathy: an update meta-analysis. Clin Res Hepatol Gastroenterol 2015;39(6): 674–82.
65. McGee RG, et al. Probiotics for patients with hepatic encephalopathy. Cochrane Database Syst Rev 2011;(11):CD008716.

Nonpharmacologic Management of Hepatic Encephalopathy: An Update

Vanessa Weir, BA[a], K. Rajender Reddy, MD[b],*

KEYWORDS

- Hepatic encephalopathy • Nonpharmacologic • Probiotics
- Fecal microbiota transplant • Nutrition • Prebiotics • Gut microbiome
- Branched-chain amino acids

KEY POINTS

- Nonpharmacologic treatments of hepatic encephalopathy (HE) target the gut-liver-brain axis, which studies increasingly show may underlie its pathophysiology.
- Metaanalyses reveal that probiotics, compared with placebo, may be beneficial in treating and preventing HE.
- Nutritional intervention remains an effective adjunct in the management of HE, although preferred protein source remains a controversial topic.
- Fecal microbiota transplants, which act by correcting gut dysbiosis, report promising results as a novel therapy for HE.
- The use of the molecular adsorbent recirculating system in HE is promising, although the data are not robust enough for recommending its ubiquitous use.

INTRODUCTION

Hepatic encephalopathy (HE) is a state of altered neurocognitive function because of a combination of spontaneous portosystemic shunting and hepatic insufficiency. It is commonly encountered in association with acute liver failure (ALF), created portosystemic shunts either surgically or radiologically (transjugular intrahepatic portosystemic shunt), and cirrhosis.[1,2] Using West Haven and International Society for Hepatic Encephalopathy and Nitrogen Metabolism criteria, it can be characterized as covert (minimal hepatic encephalopathy [MHE] and grade 1), often needing specialized testing to discern brain dysfunction, or overt (grade 2, 3, 4), which produces more

a Division of Gastroenterology and Hepatology, Department of Medicine, University of Pennsylvania, Perelman Center for Advanced Medicine, 7 South Pavilion, 3400 Civic Center Boulevard, HUP, Philadelphia, PA 19104, USA; b Division of Gastroenterology and Hepatology, Department of Medicine, University of Pennsylvania, 2 Dulles, 3400 Spruce Street, HUP, Philadelphia, PA 19104, USA
* Corresponding author.
E-mail address: Rajender.reddy@pennmedicine.upenn.edu

Clin Liver Dis 24 (2020) 243–261
https://doi.org/10.1016/j.cld.2020.01.003
1089-3261/20/© 2020 Elsevier Inc. All rights reserved.

severe symptoms that include marked disorientation, asterisks, and coma.[2] MHE affects 50% to 80% of patients with cirrhosis and is associated with impaired health-related quality of life,[3–5] whereas covert HE is associated with decreased survival rates, increased hospitalization risk, and increased risk of progression to overt hepatic encephalopathy (OHE).[6] OHE episodes affect about 30% to 45% of patients with cirrhosis in their lifetime[7,8] and are associated with worse prognosis and increased hospitalization rates.[9]

Currently, practice guidelines by the European Association for the Study of the Liver (EASL) and American Association for the Study of Liver Diseases (AASLD) recommend nonabsorbable disaccharides like lactulose and/or antibiotics like rifaximin for the treatment and secondary prophylaxis of OHE.[2] However, poor tolerability,[10] the possibility of antibiotic resistance,[11] and the prevalence of treatment resistance[12] require the investigation of alternative therapies. With emerging literature demonstrating the connection between the gut microbiome, liver, and brain,[13] it seems logical to evaluate the efficacy of HE treatments that target this axis. This review outlines the role of the microbiome in HE and evaluates the current status of emerging nonpharmacologic treatment options like probiotics, nutritional management, and fecal microbiota transplants (FMT). Furthermore, the efficacy of liver support devices and orthotopic liver transplantation (OLT) to treat HE is addressed.

PATHOPHYSIOLOGY AND CURRENT STANDARDS OF CARE

The pathophysiology of HE is hypothesized to be mediated through a combination of mechanisms,[14] including increased cerebral inflammation and neurotoxins, oxidative stress, blood-brain barrier impairment, and cerebral metabolism dysfunction, but is primarily thought to be the result of hyperammonemia[15] and systemic inflammation.[16]

Current standard-of-care (SOC) treatments consist of nonabsorbable disaccharides like lactulose (or to a lesser extent lactitol) and/or an oral antibiotic like rifaximin.[17] Lactulose prevents ammonia absorption in the colon by lowering pH through generating hydrogen ions and converting absorbable ammonia into nonabsorbable ammonium, increasing colonic transit time, and reducing bacterial ammonia production.[14,18] Although the therapeutic effects of lactulose are primarily thought to arise from its laxative effects, it also acts as a prebiotic, potentiating the growth of beneficial taxa in the gut.[19] A recent metaanalysis suggested that lactulose was beneficial for both treatment and prevention of MHE and OHE and reduced liver-related complications and mortality.[20] However, the adverse gastrointestinal effects of lactulose often lead to suboptimal adherence,[10] and overuse may promote complications, such as dehydration, hypernatremia, and poor nutritional uptake,[10] and may even perpetuate or precipitate HE.[14] Rifaximin is a nonabsorbable antibiotic that treats HE by reducing ammonia-producing flora, correcting gut dysbiosis, and decreasing inflammation.[14,18] A metaanalysis notes that rifaximin was as effective as lactulose in treating HE,[21] and combined treatment showed significant decreases in OHE compared with lactulose alone.[22] Thus, rifaximin conjunction therapy with lactulose is recommended by the EASL and AASLD guidelines for secondary prophylaxis of OHE in patients resistant to lactulose-alone therapy.[2]

THE GUT-LIVER-BRAIN CONNECTION
The Role of the Gut in Liver Diseases

A growing body of evidence has consistently demonstrated that the gut microbiome and the progression of liver diseases are well linked.[23,24] This concept is not novel, but rather seems intuitive because the liver receives about three-quarters of its blood supply from the gut through the portal vein.[24] Patients with cirrhosis exhibit measurable changes in the composition of their intestinal microbiomes,[23] including a high incidence of small intestinal bacterial overgrowth (SIBO)[25,26] and increased intestinal epithelial permeability.[27,28] These intestinal modifications are, in part, due to the association between advanced liver disease and decreased bile acid release, whose antimicrobial properties are shown to prevent intestinal bacterial overgrowth and promote intestinal epithelial barrier integrity.[29] Because the intestinal barrier serves as the primary defense mechanism to protect the liver from gut-derived pathogens,[30] increased intestinal permeability is associated with a proinflammatory response.[31,32]

In addition to decreased intestinal barrier function, gut dysbiosis, or the imbalance between helpful and harmful bacteria, is associated with increased inflammation, fibrosis, and hepatic steatosis.[33–35] In fact, patients with cirrhosis exhibit decreases in "good" autochthonous bacteria (Ruminococcaceae, Lachnospiraceae, and Clostridiales XIV)[36,37] and increases in "bad" pathogenic bacteria (Enterobacteriaceae, Enterococcaeae, Staphylococcaceae, Veillonellaceae, and Streptococcaceae),[36,37] leading to the creation of the cirrhosis dysbiosis ratio (CDR) to quantify this dysregulation.[36] Autochthonous taxa is known to be a regulator in bile acid homeostasis[38,39] and colonic mucosal immunology,[40] whereas overgrowth of pathogenic taxa is associated with endotoxemia and disease progression.[25,37,40] Because CDR ratios have been shown to decrease from healthy controls (2.05) to those with compensated cirrhosis (0.89), decompensated cirrhosis (0.66), and inpatients (0.32, $P<.0001$), the CDR ratio quantifiably indicates the association between gut dysbiosis and liver disease progression.[36]

The increased intestinal permeability associated with portal hypertension, SIBO, and gut dysbiosis leads to elevated bacterial translocation.[27,41] This migration of bacteria and recognition of bacterial-derived antigens in the liver prompt a proinflammatory liver response and systemic inflammation,[27] which are associated with progression of cirrhosis and acute-on-chronic liver failure (ACLF).[42] In a cyclic nature, bacterial translocation and gut dysbiosis are shown to increase portal hypertension,[43] resulting in a "chicken-and-egg" debate.[24] The proximate interplay between gut dysbiosis, portal hypertension, bacterial translocation, intestinal integrity, and inflammatory response in the progression of liver diseases and their complications makes targeting the gut-liver axis in the treatment of decompensated liver disease a logical choice.

The Role of the Gut in Hepatic Encephalopathy

There is a critical connection between the gut microbiota, inflammation, and HE symptoms.[44,45] Patients with cirrhosis, with both MHE and OHE, exhibit significant differences in the gut microbiome than those with no cognitive impairments.[46] In both HE and non-HE patients, autochthonous genera (Blautia, Fecalibacterium, Roseburia, and Dorea) have been associated with improved cognition and decreased inflammation, whereas overgrowth of potentially pathogenic bacteria (Enterococcus and Burkholderia) in those solely with HE has associated with attenuated cognition and potentiated inflammation.[40] Robust correlations between cognition, the microbiome (specifically Alcaligeneceae, Porphyromonadaceae, Enterobacteriaceae), and cytokines (interleukin-23 [IL-23], IL-1b, IL-2, IL-4, IL-13) have been observed exclusively in those with HE.[44] One large-scale survey revealed a significantly higher abundance of Streptococcaceae in stool microbiota in those with MHE than those without, and this positively correlated with ammonia concentration.[47] In contrast, a study by Bajaj and colleagues[36,44] showed no differences in stool microbiomes for OHE patients compared with non-OHE patients but a significant difference in the sigmoid colonic mucosal microbiomes,[36] suggesting some mechanistic actions of HE may occur at the mucosal interface rather than at the luminal interface. Taken together, this indicates even beyond liver disease progression, gut dysbiosis uniquely influences HE progression and may be associated with inflammatory mechanisms. **Fig. 1** highlights the gut-liver-brain connection in the pathophysiology of HE and shows targets for SOC and nonpharmacologic treatments.

It is important to note when comparing the microbiomes of patients with cirrhosis, those with HE often consist of patients with more progressed liver disease. Because standard medications for individuals with HE act on the gut microbiome, inclusion of those patients could be potentially confounding to analyses of microbiome composition.[46] Importantly, lactulose was not shown to affect the fecal microbiota in healthy participants.[48] Although the associations between microbiota changes and hepatic decompensations like encephalopathy are in no way indicative of causation, they provide insight into the linkage of the gut microbiome with both cognitive abilities and inflammatory response and further support targeting the gut microbiome in the treatment of HE. **Table 1** lists the current nonpharmacologic treatments of HE with their mechanisms of action and efficacies.

PROBIOTICS, PREBIOTICS, AND SYNBIOTICS

Emerging literature suggests that prebiotics, probiotics, and synbiotics may treat HE through alteration of the gut microbiome.[49] Probiotics are defined as "live microorganisms which, when administered in adequate amounts, confer a health benefit on the host."[50] The most recent definition of prebiotics defines it as "a non-digestible compound that, through its metabolization by microorganisms in the gut, modulates the composition and/or activity of the gut microbiota, thus conferring a beneficial physiological effect on the host."[51] Synbiotics are a combination of probiotics and prebiotics. The hypothesized mechanism of action of these compounds involves decreasing bacterial urease activity, ammonia absorption, intestinal permeability, and bacterial translocation to result in reduced endotoxemia and inflammation.[52] Recent metaanalyses suggest probiotics to be efficacious in treating MHE and OHE compared with placebo,[53–60] but overwhelmingly do not show increased efficacy compared with lactulose,[57–60] as shown in **Table 2**.

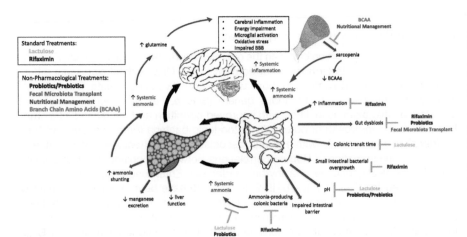

Fig. 1. Pathophysiology of HE and targets for pharmacologic and non-pharmacologic treatments. BBB, blood-brain barrier.

Table 1
Nonpharmacologic treatments of hepatic encephalopathy

Treatment Name	Stage of Development	Mechanism	Evidence	Safety	Efficacy	Recommendation
Probiotics	RCT	Correcting gut dysbiosis, reducing bacterial translocation	Cao et al,[60] 2018; Dalal et al,[59] 2017	Did not increase SAE	Probiotics could be beneficial at improving MHE and prophylaxis of OHE compared with placebo, but studies have not indicated increased efficacy over lactulose	Not yet recommended, more RCT studies needed
FMT	Phase 1 [NCT03152188] Phase 2 underway	Correcting gut dysbiosis, reducing bacterial translocation	Bajaj et al,[66] 2019	Capsular FMT had no FMT-related SAEs	FMT decreased HE recurrence, hospitalization, and improved cognitive functions, although studies were not powered for efficacy	Not yet recommended, larger-scale RCT needed
Nutritional management		Preventing degradation of skeletal muscles that detoxify ammonia		Did not increase SAE	30–35 kcal/kg/d, 1.0–1.5 g vegetable protein/kg/d significantly reversed MHE and decreased OHE development[82]	Energy intake of 35–40 kcal/kg ideal body weight, protein intake of 1.2–1.5 g/kg/d, small meals evenly distributed with a late-night snack

(continued on next page)

Table 1
(continued)

Treatment Name	Stage of Development	Mechanism	Evidence	Safety	Efficacy	Recommendation
Branched chain amino acids	RCT	Preventing degradation of skeletal muscles that detoxify ammonia	Gluud et al,[91] 2017	Did not increase SAE	Analyzed without lactulose and neomycin control, BCAA had a beneficial effect; analyzed with lactulose and neomycin, no beneficial or detrimental effect was found	Oral BCAA can be used as an alternative or additional agent to treat patients nonresponsive to conventional therapy; oral BCAA supplements can be used for patients intolerant to proteins

Abbreviations: BCAA, branched-chain amino acids; FMT, fecal microbiota transplant; MHE, minimal hepatic encephalopathy; OHE, overt hepatic encephalopathy; SAE, serious adverse events; RCT, randomized controlled trial.

Table 2
Metaanalyses of the efficacy of probiotics in treatment of hepatic encephalopathy

Study Title Date	Trials/ Patients	Groups (n)	Endpoint	Results
Shukla et al,[53] 2011	9/349	P/P/S (211) Placebo (138)	Risk of no improvement of MHE	P/P/S significantly reduced the risk of no improvement of MHE
Holte et al,[54] 2012	6/333	P/S (171) Lactulose/placebo (162)	Improvement in HE	P/S significantly improved HE
		P/S (171) Lactulose/placebo (162)	Deterioration of HE or MHE to OHE progression	NSE
Xu et al,[55] 2014	4/394	Probiotics (207) Control (187)	OHE development	Probiotics significantly reduced OHE development
Zhao et al,[56] 2015	6/450	Probiotics (229) Placebo (221)	Improvement in HE or prophylaxis of OHE	Probiotics significantly improved MHE and prophylaxis of OHE
Saab et al,[57] 2016	7/352	Probiotic (174) Placebo/no treatment (178)	MHE improvement	Probiotics significantly increased MHE improvement
	4/312	Probiotics (157) Lactulose (155)		NSE
	7/611	Probiotics (317) Placebo/no treatment (294)	MHE to OHE progression or worsening of OHE	Probiotics significantly decreased MHE to OHE progression or worsening of OHE
	6/449	Probiotics (224) Lactulose (225)		NSE
	4/316	Probiotics (169) Placebo/no treatment (147)	Prophylaxis of OHE	Probiotics significantly decreased the development of OHE
	4/291	Probiotics (146) Lactulose (145)		NSE
Viramontes Hörner et al,[58] 2017	9/570	Probiotics (308) Placebo/no treatment (262)	Reversal of MHE	Probiotics significantly reversed MHE
	4/265	Probiotics (130) Lactulose (135)		NSE
	6/587	Probiotics (303) Placebo/no treatment (284)	Development of OHE	Probiotics significantly reduced OHE development
	4/392	Probiotics (194) Lactulose (198)		NSE
Dalal et al,[59] 2017	10/574	Probiotics (293) Placebo/no treatment (281)	No recovery from HE symptoms	Probiotics significantly reduced no recovery from HE symptoms
	7/430	Probiotics (213) Lactulose (217)	Lack of recovery from HE symptoms	NSE

(continued on next page)

	Trials/			
Study Title Date	**Patients**	**Groups (n)**	**Endpoint**	**Results**
Cao et al,[60] 2018	a. 3/191 b. 3/205	Probiotics a. (96) b. (104) Placebo/no treatment a. (95) b. (101)	Prevent OHE at a. 4 wk or b. 12 wk	a. Probiotics significantly decreased OHE progression at 4 wk b. NSE
	a. 2/130 b. 2/125	Probiotics a. (66) b. (62) Lactulose a. (64) b. (63)		a. NSE b. NSE
	a. 2/131 b. 3/205	Probiotics a. (65) b. (101) Placebo/no treatment a. (66) b. (104)	Improve MHE at a. 4 wk or b. 12 wk	a. & b. Probiotics significantly improved MHE at 4 and 12 wk
	a. 2/130 b. 2/125	Probiotics a. (66) b. (62) Lactulose a. (64) b. (63)		a. NSE b. NSE
	a. 2/104 b. 2/90	Probiotics a. (54) b. (44) Placebo/no treatment a. (50) b. (46)	Improvement of NCT values in a. 4 wk or b. 8 wk	a. Probiotics decreased NCT at 4 wk b. NSE at 8 wk
	a.1/70 b. 1/44	Probiotics a. (35) b. (23) Lactulose a. (35) b. (21)		a. Lactulose significantly decreased NCT at 4 wk compared with probiotics b. NSE at 8 wk

Table 2
(continued)

Abbreviations: HE, hepatic encephalopathy; MHE, minimal hepatic encephalopathy; NCT, number connection test; NSE, no significant effect; OHE, overt hepatic encephalopathy; P/P/S, prebiotics, probiotics, and synbiotics; P/S, probiotics and synbiotics; wk, weeks.

Viramontes and colleagues[58] demonstrated that probiotics significantly reversed MHE (risk ratio [RR]: 1.53, 95% confidence interval [CI]: 1.14–2.05, $P = .005$) and reduced OHE (RR: 0.62, 95% CI: 0.48–0.80, $P = .0002$) in comparison to placebo; however, no significant effects were found when compared with lactulose. Similarly, a metaanalysis by Cao and colleagues[60] showed probiotics to be effective in treating MHE by significantly reducing number connection test score (NCT) (4 weeks) (mean difference [MD]: -30.25, 95% CI: -49.85 to -10.66, $P = .002$), preventing OHE development (4 weeks) (odds ratio [OR]: 0.22, 95% CI: 0.07–0.67, $P = .008$), and improving MHE (4 and 12 weeks) (OR: 0.18, 95% CI: 0.07–0.47, $P = .0004$ and OR: 0.15, 95% CI:

0.07–0.32, P<.00001) compared with placebo/no treatment. However, it is important to note that longer follow-up demonstrated no significant effects in reducing NCT (P = .33) or preventing OHE development (P = .09) at 8 and 12 weeks, respectively. The investigators furthermore concluded probiotics to be comparable to lactulose in improving MHE and preventing OHE, although caution should be taken when equating lack of significant effect to comparable efficacies.

A metaanalysis by Dalal and colleagues[59] similarly revealed probiotics to significantly reduce HE symptoms compared with placebo (RR 0.67, 95% CI: 0.56–0.79, P<.00001) but not lactulose. This review noted that probiotics decreased plasma ammonia concentrations (MD −8.29, 95% CI: −13.17 to −3.41, P = .000087) and may have slightly improved quality of life in comparison to no treatment, albeit with low-quality evidence. Adverse events were lower (RR 0.29, 95% CI: 0.16–0.51, P = .000024) when treated with probiotics compared with no treatment/placebo, although all-cause mortalities were not affected. In addition, very low-quality evidence prevented any decisive conclusions when comparing probiotic treatment to lactulose. The efficacy of probiotics in decreasing hospitalization rates is unclear with 1 metaanalysis showing decreased hospitalization rates compared with placebo (OR: 0.53, 95% CI: 0.33–0.86, P = .01)[57] and another demonstrating uncertain results.[59] Subanalyses of individual probiotic species from the Dalal and colleagues review and 2 additional randomized controlled trials (RCTs) revealed that *Lactobacilli*, *Bifidobacteria*, *Streptococcus thermophiles*, and VSL #3 specifically might reduce overt HE in at-risk patients and lead to improvements in MHE symptoms in comparison to placebo.[61]

Overall, probiotics seem to be safe and confer some benefit in treating and preventing HE compared with placebo, but do not appear to be more efficacious than lactulose. In addition, evidence remains uncertain if the conferred benefit of probiotics leads to reduced hospitalization and mortality. Many of these metaanalyses suffered from limitations like short-term treatment in many of the trials, nonstandardization of probiotic formulas and doses, and high risk of systematic and random error. Thus, future trials should focus on high-quality, standardized collections using both placebo and lactulose comparisons to discern the true effectiveness of probiotics to treat HE.

FECAL MICROBIOTA TRANSPLANTATION

Given that FMT have shown efficacy to correct gut dysbiosis in other conditions,[62,63] there is an increasing interest in their use to treat HE. In the first RCT conducted by Bajaj and colleagues,[64] 20 participants were randomized to a rationally selected donor FMT enema (n = 10) or control arm (n = 10) while continuing on their lactulose and rifaximin therapy. The FMT arm was given a 5-day treatment of antibiotics to promote receptivity to donor bacterial colonization and then given 1 FMT enema high in the beneficial taxa Lachnoptiacae and Ruminococcaeae. Results showed significantly fewer serious adverse events (SAEs) (P = .02) in the FMT arm (2 total, 0 liver related) than the SOC arm (11 total, 9 liver related). Six total HE episodes were observed in the SOC arm compared with 0 in the FMT arm (P = .03). In addition, there was a significant cognitive improvement in the FMT arm compared with baseline as indicated by improved psychometric hepatic encephalopathy score (PHES) (P = .003) and EncephalApp Stroop (P = .01) scores, whereas this was not seen in the SOC arm. Although improvements on these validated cognitive tests suggest a clinically meaningful impact of FMT treatment on HE, the results are limited because of sample size, short follow-up time (20 days), and antibiotic pretreatment on exclusively the FMT arm.

In a 12-month follow-up of those patients, FMT seemed safe and potentially efficacious long term.[65] There were significantly fewer hospitalizations (1 FMT, 10 SOC,

$P = .05$) and HE episodes (0 FMT, 8 SOC, $P = .03$) in the FMT arm than SOC. Similarly, cognitive function as measured by PHES ($P = .02$) and EncephalApp Stroop test ($P = .03$) remained significantly better for FMT recipients. Although there were long-term variations in FMT versus SOC stool microbiomes, Lachnospiraceae and Rumino-coccaceae relative abundances were similar between groups, which is interesting because although the donor was rich in those species, these results could indicate that the beneficial effects are not necessarily conferred through a reflection of donor microbiota. Although it is important to note that 2 SOC and 1 FMT were excluded from this follow-up (2 died, 1 OLT), this study suggests FMT may be safe and efficacious long term, although large-scale controlled trials are needed to confirm these preliminary results.

In a recent phase 1 placebo-controlled trial by Bajaj and colleagues,[66] capsular FMTs were shown to be well tolerated and safe. There was 1 reported SAE in the FMT group (n = 10) compared with 11 reported in the placebo group (n = 10, $P<.05$). Although not powered to investigate the efficacy, FMTs were associated with changes indicative of HE improvement, such as improved EncephalApp Stroop test performance ($P<.05$), although PHES did not improve. In addition, within the FMT arm, there was increased duodenal mucosal microbial diversity compared with baseline. Specifically, the duodenal microbiota showed increases in Ruminococcaeae and Bifidobacteriaceae and reductions in Steptococcaceae and Veillonellaceae. Reductions in Veillonellaceae were found in the sigmoid and stool microbiotas as well. Streptococacaeae and Veillonellacaea are often present in higher ratios in the intestinal mucosa and stool of cirrhotic patients,[23] and Streptococcaeae specifically has been linked with HE because of its expression of the ammonia-producing enzyme urease.[47] Therefore, these changes, which were also associated with favorable intestinal inflammatory responses, suggest the FMT may beneficially modulate the intestinal barrier and decrease bacterial taxa associated with the progression of cirrhosis. However, patients with HE episodes were similar between groups (placebo = 3, FMT = 1), although there was a trend toward lower hospitalizations in FMT-assigned patients (placebo = 6, FMT = 1). It is important to note both the small sample size (10 per group) and the study design limitations, including that placebo controls did not receive repeat endoscopies. Nonetheless, these promising results invoke the need for additional larger-scale placebo-controlled RCT to determine the efficacy of FMT for treatment and secondary prophylaxis of HE. Currently, phase 2 clinical trials are underway (NCT03420482) to assess the efficacy of 21 days of FMT oral capsules on neurologic function in patients with a history of HE.

DIETARY AND SUPPLEMENTAL MANAGEMENT
Energy and Protein Guidelines

Evidence shows that malnutrition correlates with HE in a relationship that seems to be linked with ammonia metabolism in the muscles.[67,68] Although historically protein restriction was hypothesized to reduce plasma ammonia levels,[69,70] studies have consistently shown no beneficial effect of dietary protein restriction and even observed this practice to contribute to detrimental muscle wasting, also known as sarcopenia.[71,72] Because the muscles are a major site of ammonia detoxification, especially in patients with cirrhosis,[73] decreases in muscle mass are associated with an increased incidence of HE.[74] Thus, nutritional guidelines to prevent muscle wasting are relevant in the prevention and treatment of HE. In the effort to minimize muscle depletion, nutritional recommendations centralize around reducing gluconeogenesis, which depletes muscles by using amino acids to produce glucose for fuel. Patients are recommended minimum calorie and protein intake suggestions and are advised to avoid fasting by eating small, frequent meals[75] and by consuming a late-night snack.[76] Current EASL and AASLD guidelines recommend that caloric intake should be 35 to 40 kcal/kg of ideal body weight with 1.2 to 1.5 g/kg protein per day.[2] With the increasing epidemic of overweight and obese patients with cirrhosis,[77] it is essential to also ensure the required caloric and protein intake in this unique population to avoid muscle breakdown while concurrently trying to reduce body weight.[75] In addition, studies have shown that hyponatremia, likely dilutional in nature, is a risk factor for HE in patients with cirrhosis.[78] Therefore, is it recommended that sodium intake and water balance be monitored in patients with a history of HE episodes as well.[75]

The source of dietary protein remains a cause of contention within the medical community. Bianchi and colleagues[79] showed that the adjunct of a plant-based therapy to be uniquely beneficial in decreasing HE grade, increasing performance on psychometric tests, and decreasing fasting ammonia levels compared with an isonitrogenous animal protein diet. It is hypothesized that the mechanism underlying these differences could be due to increased branched-chain amino acids (BCAA) and decreased mercaptan formation.[80] However, a less-explored potential mechanism is the increased availability of fermentable fibers, which act as a prebiotic "natural lactulose" to lower colonic pH and increase ammonia/ammonium excretion.[71] Additional studies have found contradictory evidence by showing no significant difference in symptom recovery between vegetable and animal protein for HE patients.[81] Also, the decreased palatability of plant-based diets could make patient compliance an issue.[81] Future clinical trials should aim to examine the effect of an increased fermentable fiber diet on the progression of HE in addition to the current nutritional management guidelines.

In a recent RCT evaluating the efficacy of nutritional management in MHE treatment, nutritional therapy of 30 to 35 kcal/kg with 1.0 to 1.5 g/kg ideal body weight of vegetable protein was shown to significantly reverse MHE (71.1% vs 22.8%; $P = .001$) and decrease OHE development (10% vs 21.7%; $P = .04$) after 6 months. In addition, patients had increases in PHES scores (3.86 ± 3.58 vs 0.52 ± 4.09; $P = .001$) and health-related quality-of-life scores (3.24 ± 3.63 vs 0.54 ± 3.58; $P = .001$).[82] However, Child-Pugh class C patients did not achieve the same degree of improvement as Child-Pugh class B, indicating that nutritional management may be better therapeutically for less decompensated patients. Although some evidence points out that nutritional support may not confer any direct benefit to liver diseases,[83] this study suggests that nutritional management could be beneficial in decreasing some of its complications, like MHE progression. Taken together, nutritional management of HE is relevant as an adjunct therapy, although future studies should aim to delineate specific energy balance criteria for overweight and obese patients as well as to determine if there are unique benefits for specific protein sources.

Branched-Chain Amino Acids

BCAAs (valine, leucine, and isoleucine) are amino acids initially metabolized in the skeletal muscle instead of the liver.[84] Skeletal muscles are a major site of ammonia detoxification in patients with cirrhosis,[73] and studies show that muscle BCAA may be implicated in ammonia removal.[85] In the presence of protein-energy malnutrition, patients with cirrhosis become hyperglucagonemic, which leads to increased utilization of BCAA by skeletal muscles for resynthesis of glutamine, an essential component for ammonia clearance in liver-deficient patients.[86] In addition, reduced plasma BCAAs in patients with cirrhosis was associated with high levels of aromatic amino acids, a relationship called a Fischer's ratio, and was shown to correlate with HE grade.[87] Thus, it is hypothesized that BCAA supplementation could treat HE by reducing muscle loss,[88,89] increasing ammonia detoxification via glutamine synthesis,[88] and decreasing influx of aromatic amino acids across the blood-brain barrier.[90]

In a recent Cochrane metaanalysis, BCAA had a beneficial effect on HE, with no increased risk of SAEs.[91] However, more trials were needed to determine its efficacy compared with SOC treatments like lactulose and rifaximin. Currently, EASL and AASLD guidelines recommend oral BCAA as an alternative therapy for the treatment of nonresponsive OHE patients as well as to supplement nitrogen intake for protein-intolerant individuals.[2]

PROCEDURAL TREATMENT OF HEPATIC ENCEPHALOPATHY

HE is a common manifestation in patients progressing to liver failure, including those with ALF, ACLF, and end-stage liver disease, and its presence is associated with increased mortality.[9] When a declining liver condition necessitates an OLT as the remaining therapeutic option, extracorporeal liver support devices (ELSD) have shown promise as a supportive treatment in those with declining liver function when transplantation options are unavailable.[92]

Liver Support Devices

ELSD act to provide temporary liver function by removing toxins from the blood until suitable liver regeneration or organ transplantation is available.[93] One current ELSD device is artificial liver support (ALS), which facilitates removal of liver toxins through cell-free techniques and includes those based on conventional procedures as well as those using albumin dialysis (ie, molecular adsorbent recirculating system [MARS]). In addition, biological extracorporeal liver perfusion is a type of ELSD using animal or human livers, and bioartificial liver support is a hybrid system using liver cells.[92]

Although standard dialysis techniques, such as hemodialysis, cannot remove protein-bound molecules, they are effective at removal of ammonia and urea.[94] A retrospective study (n = 340) showed continuous renal replacement therapy, but not intermittent renal replacement therapy, to decrease serum ammonia levels and mortality in ALF.[95] Albumin dialysis removes albumin-bound toxins in addition to water-soluble molecules like cytokines, ammonia, and urea. One of the most readily used ALS using albumin dialysis in HE treatment is the MARS.[96] It contains 3 circuits: blood, albumin, and dialysate, using dialysate that is regenerated via charcoal and an anion resin recirculated in a 6- to 8-hour session.[97,98] In patients with ACLF, a metaanalysis showed that MARS treatment resulted in a significant improvement in HE grade (P<.001).[99] Furthermore, a prospective RCT in patients with cirrhosis (n = 70) exhibiting grade III or IV HE revealed a higher improvement proportion of HE in the standard medical therapy (SMT) + MARS group than those receiving SMT alone (P<.044), although treatment was only for 5 days, so effects on survival or long-term efficacy could not be assessed.[100] Similarly, the RELIEF study (n = 189) found MARS to decrease HE grade compared with SMT alone (P = .07), but conferred no benefit on survival rates in patients with ACLF.[101] In a study of patients with ALF, an RCT found that HE did not improve in a clinically significant way following MARS treatment.[102]

Liver Transplantation

In the case of persistent OHE, correcting the underlying liver dysfunction via OLT may be the final therapeutic option. However, although severe HE (grade 3–4) has been shown to correlate with increased waitlist mortality in patients with model for end-stage liver disease (MELD) ≥30,[103] HE does not factor into MELD score, and thus waitlist priority, for liver transplant recipients. The degree to which OLT can fully restore cognitive function remains somewhat controversial. Following a liver transplant, patients with MHE showed persistent improvements in cognitive function, including visuospatial and selective attention, visuospatial short- and long-term memory, and language tasks after 6 months,[104] but vasomotor deficits persisted.[105] Patients with OHE history showed normalized electroencephalograms and greater cognitive improvements after OLT, but global cognitive function remained inferior to HE-negative transplant recipients.[106] Nevertheless, between 13% and 47% of OLT recipients face neurologic complications after the procedure,[107] and these are most severe in patients with OHE episodes pre-OLT.[108] Furthermore, HE is the most commonly reported neurologic complication from OLT, although postoperative incidences range from 12% to 84%.[109] One could speculate as to whether the reported persistence of HE after transplant is actually recurrent HE or caused by the toxicity of immunosuppressants, ischemic brain injury, or persistence of portosystemic shunts.[110]

Nevertheless, the presence of preoperative HE has been shown to affect posttransplant outcomes because the stress of the procedure itself may trigger cognitive dysfunction.[111] For example, preoperative HE was the strongest predictor of posttransplant morbidities, including HE, seizures, and drug-related neurotoxicity.[111] A recent study showed that sequelae of HE post-OLT were only significantly associated with grade 3 to 4 HE before transplant but not grade 1 or 2.[112] Taken together, correcting HE development before transplant may improve posttransplant outcomes, but the data are not clear on the full reversibility of HE and thus the ability of OLT to completely treat it.

SUMMARY AND FUTURE DIRECTIONS

Emerging evidence notes the relevance of the gut microbiome-liver axis and its contribution to the pathophysiology of HE. Guidelines from EASL and AASLD have well addressed the treatment and secondary prophylaxis of OHE, although they are evolving concepts and treatment for MHE; furthermore, they do not make recommendations for the use of nonpharmacologic treatments given the controversial nature and the lack of robust data. Regardless, although evidence has not shown the increased efficacy of probiotics or nutritional management over lactulose and/or rifaximin therapies, the safety and efficacy profiles indicated via recent metaanalyses suggest probiotics could be useful in the treatment of MHE and potentially primary prophylaxis of HE in at-risk individuals. There is a need for additional large-scale, low-bias RCTs to confirm the true efficacy and safety of probiotics in the treatment of HE. Furthermore, preliminary and phase 1 trials of enema delivery and capsular FMT seem to produce promising results for HE treatment. However, outcomes from phase 2 trials will help to discern if FMT could be a viable option for the treatment and prevention of HE. Final options to treat persistent OHE include liver support devices and liver transplants, although the full reversibility of HE even after OLT is not clear. Taken together, correcting gut dysbiosis in patients with cirrhosis through administration of probiotics and rationally selected FMT could be potential therapies for the treatment and prevention of HE, although more evidence is needed to justify their use.

DISCLOSURE

K.R. Reddy: Scientific Advisory Board, L Abbvie, Gilead, Merck, Shionogi, Dova; Research Support (paid to the University of Pennsylvania): Abbvie, Merck, Gilead, Conatus, Intercept, Mallinckrodt. V. Weir: No conflicts to report.

REFERENCES

1. Blei AT, Córdoba J, Practice Parameters Committee of the American College of Gastroenterology. Hepatic encephalopathy. Am J Gastroenterol 2001;96(7): 1968–76.
2. Vilstrup H, Amodio P, Bajaj J, et al. Hepatic encephalopathy in chronic liver disease: 2014 practice guideline by the American Association for the Study of Liver Diseases and the European Association for the Study of the Liver. Hepatology 2014;60(2):715–35.
3. Bajaj JS, Saeian K, Verber MD, et al. Inhibitory control test is a simple method to diagnose minimal hepatic encephalopathy and predict development of overt hepatic encephalopathy. Am J Gastroenterol 2007;102(4):754–60.
4. Das A, Dhiman RK, Saraswat VA, et al. Prevalence and natural history of subclinical hepatic encephalopathy in cirrhosis. J Gastroenterol Hepatol 2001;16(5): 531–5.
5. Bale A, Pai CG, Shetty S, et al. Prevalence of and factors associated with minimal hepatic encephalopathy in patients with cirrhosis of liver. J Clin Exp Hepatol 2018;8(2):156–61.
6. Patidar KR, Thacker LR, Wade JB, et al. Covert hepatic encephalopathy is independently associated with poor survival and increased risk of hospitalization. Am J Gastroenterol 2014;109(11):1757–63.
7. Romero-Gómez M, Boza F, García-Valdecasas MS, et al. Subclinical hepatic encephalopathy predicts the development of overt hepatic encephalopathy. Am J Gastroenterol 2001;96(9):2718–23.
8. Poordad FF. Review article: the burden of hepatic encephalopathy. Aliment Pharmacol Ther 2007;25(Suppl 1):3–9.
9. Cordoba J, Ventura-Cots M, Simón-Talero M, et al. Characteristics, risk factors, and mortality of cirrhotic patients hospitalized for hepatic encephalopathy with and without acute-on-chronic liver failure (ACLF). J Hepatol 2014;60(2):275–81.
10. Bajaj JS, Sanyal AJ, Bell D, et al. Predictors of the recurrence of hepatic encephalopathy in lactulose-treated patients. Aliment Pharmacol Ther 2010;31(9): 1012–7.
11. O'Connor JR, Galang MA, Sambol SP, et al. Rifampin and rifaximin resistance in clinical isolates of Clostridium difficile. Antimicrob Agents Chemother 2008; 52(8):2813–7.
12. Bajaj JS, Schubert CM, Heuman DM, et al. Persistence of cognitive impairment after resolution of overt hepatic encephalopathy. Gastroenterology 2010;138(7): 2332–40.
13. Mancini A, Campagna F, Amodio P, et al. Gut : liver : brain axis: the microbial challenge in the hepatic encephalopathy. Food Funct 2018;9(3):1373–88.
14. Hadjihambi A, Arias N, Sheikh M, et al. Hepatic encephalopathy: a critical current review. Hepatol Int 2018;12(Suppl 1):135–47.
15. Wijdicks EF. Hepatic encephalopathy. N Engl J Med 2016;375(17):1660–70.
16. Tranah T, Vijay G, Ryan J, et al. Systemic inflammation and ammonia in hepatic encephalopathy. Metab Brain Dis 2013;28(1):1–5.
17. Bajaj JS. Hepatic encephalopathy: classification and treatment. J Hepatol 2018; 68(4):838–9.
18. Swaminathan M, Ellul MA, Cross TJ. Hepatic encephalopathy: current challenges and future prospects. Hepat Med 2018;10:1–11.
19. De Preter V, Vanhoutte T, Huys G, et al. Effect of lactulose and Saccharomyces boulardii administration on the colonic urea-nitrogen metabolism and the

bifidobacteria concentration in healthy human subjects. Aliment Pharmacol Ther 2006;23(7):963–74.

20. Gluud LL, Vilstrup H, Morgan MY. Nonabsorbable disaccharides for hepatic encephalopathy: a systematic review and meta-analysis. Hepatology 2016;64(3): 908–22.

21. Wu D, Wu SM, Lu J, et al. Rifaximin versus nonabsorbable disaccharides for the treatment of hepatic encephalopathy: a meta-analysis. Gastroenterol Res Pract 2013;2013:236963.

22. Sharma BC, Sharma P, Lunia MK, et al. A randomized, double-blind, controlled trial comparing rifaximin plus lactulose with lactulose alone in treatment of overt hepatic encephalopathy. Am J Gastroenterol 2013;108(9):1458–63.

23. Qin N, Yang F, Li A, et al. Alterations of the human gut microbiome in liver cirrhosis. Nature 2014;513(7516):59–64.

24. Arab JP, Martin-Mateos RM, Shah VH. Gut-liver axis, cirrhosis and portal hypertension: the chicken and the egg. Hepatol Int 2018;12(Suppl 1):24–33.

25. Quigley EM, Stanton C, Murphy EF. The gut microbiota and the liver. Pathophysiological and clinical implications. J Hepatol 2013;58(5):1020–7.

26. Bauer TM, Steinbrückner B, Brinkmann FE, et al. Small intestinal bacterial overgrowth in patients with cirrhosis: prevalence and relation with spontaneous bacterial peritonitis. Am J Gastroenterol 2001;96(10):2962–7.

27. Wiest R, Garcia-Tsao G. Bacterial translocation (BT) in cirrhosis. Hepatology 2005;41(3):422–33.

28. Pijls KE, Jonkers DM, Elamin EE, et al. Intestinal epithelial barrier function in liver cirrhosis: an extensive review of the literature. Liver Int 2013;33(10):1457–69.

29. Cariou B, Staels B. The expanding role of the bile acid receptor FXR in the small intestine. J Hepatol 2006;44(6):1213–5.

30. Marchiando A, Graham W, Turner J. Epithelial barriers in homeostasis and disease. Annu Rev Pathol 2010;5:119–44.

31. Pradere JP, Troeger JS, Dapito DH, et al. Toll-like receptor 4 and hepatic fibrogenesis. Semin Liver Dis 2010;30(3):232–44.

32. Fukui H. Increased intestinal permeability and decreased barrier function: does it really influence the risk of inflammation? Inflamm Intest Dis 2016;1(3):135–45.

33. Seki E, Schnabl B. Role of innate immunity and the microbiota in liver fibrosis: crosstalk between the liver and gut. J Physiol 2012;590(3):447–58.

34. Henao-Mejia J, Elinav E, Jin C, et al. Inflammasome-mediated dysbiosis regulates progression of NAFLD and obesity. Nature 2012;482(7384):179–85.

35. Tripathi A, Debelius J, Brenner DA, et al. The gut-liver axis and the intersection with the microbiome. Nat Rev Gastroenterol Hepatol 2018;15(7):397–411.

36. Bajaj JS, Heuman DM, Hylemon PB, et al. Altered profile of human gut microbiome is associated with cirrhosis and its complications. J Hepatol 2014; 60(5):940–7.

37. Chen Y, Yang F, Lu H, et al. Characterization of fecal microbial communities in patients with liver cirrhosis. Hepatology 2011;54(2):562–72.

38. Acharya C, Bajaj JS. Altered microbiome in patients with cirrhosis and complications. Clin Gastroenterol Hepatol 2019;17(2):307–21.

39. Schnabl B, Brenner DA. Interactions between the intestinal microbiome and liver diseases. Gastroenterology 2014;146(6):1513–24.

40. Bajaj JS, Hylemon PB, Ridlon JM, et al. Colonic mucosal microbiome differs from stool microbiome in cirrhosis and hepatic encephalopathy and is linked to cognition and inflammation. Am J Physiol Gastrointest Liver Physiol 2012; 303(6):G675–85.

41. Seo YS, Shah VH. The role of gut-liver axis in the pathogenesis of liver cirrhosis and portal hypertension. Clin Mol Hepatol 2012;18(4):337–46.

42. Bernardi M, Moreau R, Angeli P, et al. Mechanisms of decompensation and organ failure in cirrhosis: from peripheral arterial vasodilation to systemic inflammation hypothesis. J Hepatol 2015;63(5):1272–84.

43. Wiest R, Das S, Cadelina G, et al. Bacterial translocation in cirrhotic rats stimulates eNOS-derived NO production and impairs mesenteric vascular contractility. J Clin Invest 1999;104(9):1223–33.

44. Bajaj JS, Ridlon JM, Hylemon PB, et al. Linkage of gut microbiome with cognition in hepatic encephalopathy. Am J Physiol Gastrointest Liver Physiol 2012; 302(1):G168–75.

45. Rai R, Saraswat VA, Dhiman RK. Gut microbiota: its role in hepatic encephalopathy. J Clin Exp Hepatol 2015;5(Suppl 1):S29–36.

46. Bajaj JS. The role of microbiota in hepatic encephalopathy. Gut Microbes 2014; 5(3):397–403.

47. Zhang Z, Zhai H, Geng J, et al. Large-scale survey of gut microbiota associated with MHE via 16S rRNA-based pyrosequencing. Am J Gastroenterol 2013; 108(10):1601–11.

48. Vanhoutte T, De Preter V, De Brandt E, et al. Molecular monitoring of the fecal microbiota of healthy human subjects during administration of lactulose and Saccharomyces boulardii. Appl Environ Microbiol 2006;72(9):5990–7.

49. Sharma BC, Singh J. Probiotics in management of hepatic encephalopathy. Metab Brain Dis 2016;31(6):1295–301.

50. Hill C, Guarner F, Reid G, et al. Expert consensus document. The International Scientific Association for Probiotics and Prebiotics consensus statement on the scope and appropriate use of the term probiotic. Nat Rev Gastroenterol Hepatol 2014;11(8):506–14.

51. Bindels LB, Delzenne NM, Cani PD, et al. Towards a more comprehensive concept for prebiotics. Nat Rev Gastroenterol Hepatol 2015;12(5):303–10.

52. Dhiman RK. Gut microbiota and hepatic encephalopathy. Metab Brain Dis 2013; 28(2):321–6.

53. Shukla S, Shukla A, Mehboob S, et al. Meta-analysis: the effects of gut flora modulation using prebiotics, probiotics and synbiotics on minimal hepatic encephalopathy. Aliment Pharmacol Ther 2011;33(6):662–71.

54. Holte K, Krag A, Gluud LL. Systematic review and meta-analysis of randomized trials on probiotics for hepatic encephalopathy. Hepatol Res 2012;42(10): 1008–15.

55. Xu J, Ma R, Chen LF, et al. Effects of probiotic therapy on hepatic encephalopathy in patients with liver cirrhosis: an updated meta-analysis of six randomized controlled trials. Hepatobiliary Pancreat Dis Int 2014;13(4):354–60.

56. Zhao LN, Yu T, Lan SY, et al. Probiotics can improve the clinical outcomes of hepatic encephalopathy: an update meta-analysis. Clin Res Hepatol Gastroenterol 2015;39(6):674–82.

57. Saab S, Suraweera D, Au J, et al. Probiotics are helpful in hepatic encephalopathy: a meta-analysis of randomized trials. Liver Int 2016;36(7):986–93.

58. Viramontes Hörner D, Avery A, Stow R. The effects of probiotics and symbiotics on risk factors for hepatic encephalopathy: a systematic review. J Clin Gastroenterol 2017;51(4):312–23.

59. Dalal R, McGee RG, Riordan SM, et al. Probiotics for people with hepatic encephalopathy. Cochrane Database Syst Rev 2017;(2):CD008716.

60. Cao Q, Yu CB, Yang SG, et al. Effect of probiotic treatment on cirrhotic patients with minimal hepatic encephalopathy: a meta-analysis. Hepatobiliary Pancreat Dis Int 2018;17(1):9–16.

61. Koretz RL. Probiotics in gastroenterology: how pro is the evidence in adults? Am J Gastroenterol 2018;113(8):1125–36.

62. van Nood E, Vrieze A, Nieuwdorp M, et al. Duodenal infusion of donor feces for recurrent Clostridium difficile. N Engl J Med 2013;368(5):407–15.

63. Moayyedi P, Surette MG, Kim PT, et al. Fecal microbiota transplantation induces remission in patients with active ulcerative colitis in a randomized controlled trial. Gastroenterology 2015;149(1):102–9.e6.

64. Bajaj JS, Kassam Z, Fagan A, et al. Fecal microbiota transplant from a rational stool donor improves hepatic encephalopathy: a randomized clinical trial. Hepatology 2017;66(6):1727–38.

65. Bajaj JS, Fagan A, Gavis EA, et al. Long-term outcomes of fecal microbiota transplantation in patients with cirrhosis. Gastroenterology 2019;156(6): 1921–3.e3.

66. Bajaj JS, Salzman NH, Acharya C, et al. Fecal microbial transplant capsules are safe in hepatic encephalopathy: a phase 1, randomized, placebo-controlled trial. Hepatology 2019;70(5):1690–703.

67. Merli M, Iebba V, Giusto M. What is new about diet in hepatic encephalopathy. Metab Brain Dis 2016;31(6):1289–94.

68. Lattanzi B, D'Ambrosio D, Merli M. Hepatic encephalopathy and sarcopenia: two faces of the same metabolic alteration. J Clin Exp Hepatol 2019;9(1): 125–30.

69. Riordan SM, Williams R. Treatment of hepatic encephalopathy. N Engl J Med 1997;337(7):473–9.

70. Balo J, Korpassy B. The encephalitis of dogs with Eck fistula fed on meat. Arch Pathol 1932;13:80–7.

71. Yao C, Fung J, Chu N, et al. Dietary interventions in liver cirrhosis. J Clin Gastroenterol 2018;52(8):663–73.

72. Cordoba J, Lopez-Hellin J, Planas M, et al. Normal protein diet for episodic hepatic encephalopathy: results of a randomized study. J Hepatol 2004;41(1): 38–43.

73. Damink S, Deutz N, Dejong C, et al. Interorgan ammonia metabolism in liver failure. Neurochem Int 2002;41(2–3):177–88.

74. Merli M, Giusto M, Lucidi C, et al. Muscle depletion increases the risk of overt and minimal hepatic encephalopathy: results of a prospective study. Metab Brain Dis 2013;28(2):281–4.

75. Amodio P, Bemeur C, Butterworth R, et al. The nutritional management of hepatic encephalopathy in patients with cirrhosis: International Society for Hepatic Encephalopathy and Nitrogen Metabolism consensus. Hepatology 2013;58(1): 325–36.

76. Tsien CD, McCullough AJ, Dasarathy S. Late evening snack: exploiting a period of anabolic opportunity in cirrhosis. J Gastroenterol Hepatol 2012;27(3):430–41.

77. Marchesini G, Moscatiello S, Di Domizio S, et al. Obesity-associated liver disease. J Clin Endocrinol Metab 2008;93(11 Suppl 1):S74–80.

78. Guevara M, Baccaro ME, Torre A, et al. Hyponatremia is a risk factor of hepatic encephalopathy in patients with cirrhosis: a prospective study with time-dependent analysis. Am J Gastroenterol 2009;104(6):1382–9.

79. Bianchi G, Marchesini G, Fabbri A, et al. Vegetable versus animal protein-diet in cirrhotic-patients with chronic encephalopathy - a randomized cross-over comparison. J Intern Med 1993;233(5):385–92.

80. Abdelsayed GG. Diets in encephalopathy. Clin Liver Dis 2015;19(3):497–505.

81. Shaw S, Worner T, Lieber C. Comparison of animal and vegetable protein-sources in the dietary-management of hepatic-encephalopathy. Gastroenterology 1983;84(5):1396.

82. Maharshi S, Sharma BC, Sachdeva S, et al. Efficacy of nutritional therapy for patients with cirrhosis and minimal hepatic encephalopathy in a randomized trial. Clin Gastroenterol Hepatol 2016;14(3):454–60.e3 [quiz: e433].

83. Koretz RL. The evidence for the use of nutritional support in liver disease. Curr Opin Gastroenterol 2014;30(2):208–14.

84. Adibi S. Metabolism of branched-chain amino-acids in altered nutrition. Metabolism 1976;25(11):1287–302.

85. Hayashi M, Ohnishi H, Kawade Y, et al. Augmented utilization of branched-chain amino acids by skeletal muscle in decompensated liver cirrhosis in special relation to ammonia detoxication. Gastroenterol Jpn 1981;16(1):64–70.

86. Moriwaki H, Miwa Y, Tajika M, et al. Branched-chain amino acids as a protein- and energy-source in liver cirrhosis. Biochem Biophys Res Commun 2004; 313(2):405–9.

87. Fischer JE, Rosen HM, Ebeid AM, et al. The effect of normalization of plasma amino acids on hepatic encephalopathy in man. Surgery 1976;80(1):77–91.

88. Higuchi N, Kato M, Miyazaki M, et al. Potential role of branched-chain amino acids in glucose metabolism through the accelerated induction of the glucose-sensing apparatus in the liver. J Cell Biochem 2011;112(1):30–8.

89. Hiraoka A, Michitaka K, Kiguchi D, et al. Efficacy of branched-chain amino acid supplementation and walking exercise for preventing sarcopenia in patients with liver cirrhosis. Eur J Gastroenterol Hepatol 2017;29(12):1416–23.

90. Holecek M. Three targets of branched-chain amino acid supplementation in the treatment of liver disease. Nutrition 2010;26(5):482–90.

91. Gluud LL, Dam G, Les I, et al. Branched-chain amino acids for people with hepatic encephalopathy. Cochrane Database Syst Rev 2017;(5):CD001939.

92. Baquerizo A, Bañares R, Foaouzi S. Current clinical status of the extracorporeal liver support devices. In: Busuttil RW, Klintmalm GBG, editors. Transplantation of the liver. 3rd edition. Philadelphia: Elsevier Inc.; 2015. p. 1463–87.

93. Nyberg SL. Bridging the gap: advances in artificial liver support. Liver Transpl 2012;18(Suppl 2):S10–4.

94. Leckie P, Davenport A, Jalan R. Extracorporeal liver support. Blood Purif 2012; 34(2):158–63.

95. Cardoso FS, Gottfried M, Tujios S, et al. Continuous renal replacement therapy is associated with reduced serum ammonia levels and mortality in acute liver failure. Hepatology 2018;67(2):711–20.

96. Kobashi-Margain RA, Gavilanes-Espinar JG, Gutierrez-Grobe Y, et al. Albumin dialysis with molecular adsorbent recirculating system (MARS) for the treatment of hepatic encephalopathy in liver failure. Ann Hepatol 2011;10(Suppl 2):S70–6.

97. Stange J, Mitzner S, Ramlow W, et al. A new procedure for the removal of protein bound drugs and toxins. ASAIO J 1993;39(3):M621–5.

98. Kapoor D. Molecular adsorbent recirculating system: albumin dialysis-based extracorporeal liver assist device. J Gastroenterol Hepatol 2002;17(Suppl 3): S280–6.

99. Vaid A, Chweich H, Balk EM, et al. Molecular adsorbent recirculating system as artificial support therapy for liver failure: a meta-analysis. ASAIO J 2012; 58(1):51–9.

100. Hassanein TI, Tofteng F, Brown RS Jr, et al. Randomized controlled study of extracorporeal albumin dialysis for hepatic encephalopathy in advanced cirrhosis. Hepatology 2007;46(6):1853–62.

101. Banares R, Nevens F, Larsen FS, et al. Extracorporeal albumin dialysis with the molecular adsorbent recirculating system in acute-on-chronic liver failure: the RELIEF trial. Hepatology 2013;57(3):1153–62.

102. Saliba F, Camus C, Durand F, et al. Albumin dialysis with a noncell artificial liver support device in patients with acute liver failure: a randomized, controlled trial. Ann Intern Med 2013;159(8):522–31.

103. Gadiparthi C, Cholankeril G, Yoo ER, et al. Waitlist outcomes in liver transplant candidates with high MELD and severe hepatic encephalopathy. Dig Dis Sci 2018;63(6):1647–53.

104. Mattarozzi K, Stracciari A, Vignatelli L, et al. Minimal hepatic encephalopathy: longitudinal effects of liver transplantation. Arch Neurol 2004;61(2):242–7.

105. Mechtcheriakov S, Graziadei IW, Mattedi M, et al. Incomplete improvement of visuo-motor deficits in patients with minimal hepatic encephalopathy after liver transplantation. Liver Transpl 2004;10(1):77–83.

106. Campagna F, Montagnese S, Schiff S, et al. Cognitive impairment and electro-encephalographic alterations before and after liver transplantation: what is reversible? Liver Transpl 2014;20(8):977–86.

107. Stracciari A, Guarino M. Neuropsychiatric complications of liver transplantation. Metab Brain Dis 2001;16(1–2):3–11.

108. Sotil EU, Gottstein J, Ayala E, et al. Impact of preoperative overt hepatic encephalopathy on neurocognitive function after liver transplantation. Liver Transpl 2009;15(2):184–92.

109. Teperman LW. Impact of pretransplant hepatic encephalopathy on liver post-transplantation outcomes. Int J Hepatol 2013;2013:952828.

110. Atluri DK, Asgeri M, Mullen KD. Reversibility of hepatic encephalopathy after liver transplantation. Metab Brain Dis 2010;25(1):111–3.

111. Dhar R, Young GB, Marotta P. Perioperative neurological complications after liver transplantation are best predicted by pre-transplant hepatic encephalopathy. Neurocrit Care 2008;8(2):253–8.

112. You DD, Choi GS, Kim JM, et al. Long-term outcomes for liver transplant recipients in terms of hepatic encephalopathy. Transplant Proc 2017;49(6):1425–9.

The Health Care Burden of Hepatic Encephalopathy

Mohamed I. Elsaid, PhD, MPH, ALM[a],*, Tina John, MD, MPH[a], You Li, MS[a],
Sri Ram Pentakota, MD, MPH, PhD[b], Vinod K. Rustgi, MD, MBA[c]

KEYWORDS

- Hepatic encephalopathy • Economic burden • Health care costs
- Health care resource use

KEY POINTS

- Hepatic encephalopathy is neuropsychiatric complication of liver disease, which poses a significant economic and use burdens to patients and their caregivers.
- In the United States, hepatic encephalopathy accounts for 0.33% of all inpatient admissions; hepatic encephalopathy–related hospital discharges have increased by 117.7% from 2000 to 2014.
- The increase in hepatic encephalopathy–related hospitalizations translated into an increase of 197.2% in hospital charges between 2000 and 2015.
- Hepatic encephalopathy has been associated with longer inpatient length of stay, high risk of hospital readmissions, and poorer health-related quality of life compared to patients with chronic liver disease.
- Rifaximin plus lactulose has been shown in some studies to decrease the cost and health care use burdens of hepatic encephalopathy when compared with lactulose alone.

BACKGROUND

Chronic liver diseases are significant risk factors for morbidity and mortality.[1] On a global scale, chronic liver diseases affect an estimated 844 million individuals and are responsible for 2 million deaths annually, 1 million of which are related to cirrhosis and its complications.[1,2] In the United States, the use and cost burden of cirrhosis and its complications doubled between 2001 and 2011[3] and such burdens continued to increase over recent years.[4] Hepatic encephalopathy is a major neuropsychiatric

[a] Department of Medicine, Division of Gastroenterology and Hepatology, Rutgers Robert Wood Johnson Medical School, Medical Education Building, 1 Robert Wood Johnson, Room 479, New Brunswick, NJ 08903, USA; [b] Department of Surgery, Rutgers New Jersey Medical School, 185 South Orange Avenue, MSB, H-578, Newark, NJ 07101, USA; [c] Department of Medicine, Division of Gastroenterology and Hepatology, Rutgers Robert Wood Johnson Medical School, MedEd Building, Room 466, One Robert Wood Johnson Place, New Brunswick, NJ 08901, USA
* Corresponding author.
E-mail address: mie10@sph.rutgers.edu

Clin Liver Dis 24 (2020) 263–275
https://doi.org/10.1016/j.cld.2020.01.006
1089-3261/20/© 2020 Elsevier Inc. All rights reserved.

complication of liver disease and it affects 30% to 40% of cirrhotic patients.[5] Hepatic encephalopathy is characterized by a brain dysfunction that is associated with a number of neurologic complications.[5] Such neurologic complications result in cognitive impairments, which adversely affect patients' physical and mental health. In turn, hepatic encephalopathy is associated with substantial economic and use burdens to patients and their caregiver(s). Such burdens continued to increase during recent years.[6] In this review article, we aimed to provide an overview of the multidimensional aspects of the health care burden associated with hepatic encephalopathy.

EMERGENCY DEPARTMENT BURDEN

Hepatic encephalopathy is associated with significantly high health care cost and use burdens related to emergency department (ED) visits. In the United States, the overall rate of hepatic encephalopathy–related ED visits have been steadily increasing during recent years (**Fig. 1**). According to data from the Healthcare Cost and Utilization Project, the number of hepatic encephalopathy–related ED visits has significantly increased from 42,652 visits in 2006 to 57,578 in 2014.[7] The average number of ED visits with hepatic encephalopathy as the principal diagnosis during this period was 46,877. The proportion of hepatic encephalopathy visits that were discharged from the ED has increased from 11.1% in 2006 to 14.8% in 2014. During the same period, the rates of ED visits per 100,000 persons ranged between 13.2 and 18.1 in 2008 and 2014, respectively. The increase in the rates and number of visits were coupled with a significant increase in hepatic encephalopathy–related ED charges from $1357 in 2006 to $2858 in 2014.[8]

Aside from the direct burdens associated with ED visits, a significant number of patients with hepatic encephalopathy are admitted to the same hospital, whereas others continue to seek medical care in nursing homes and rehabilitation facilities. Namely, of all hepatic encephalopathy–related ED visits between 2006 and 2014, an average of 86.9% resulted in an admission to the same hospital.[7] During the

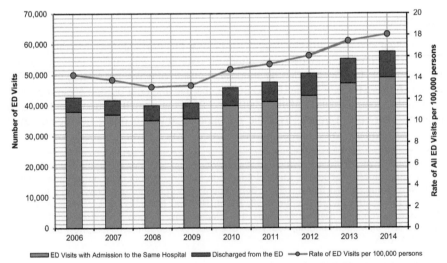

Fig. 1. Number and rates of ED visits related to hepatic encephalopathy in the United States, Nationwide Emergency Department Sample 2006 to 2014. (*Data from* the HCUPnet, Healthcare Cost and Utilization Project. Agency for Healthcare Research and Quality, Rockville, MD. https://hcupnet.ahrq.gov/.)

same period, 60.6% of all patients with hepatic encephalopathy who visited the ED and were not admitted to the same hospital had a routine discharge, whereas 8.4% were released to nursing homes or rehabilitation facilities and 24.7% were transferred to another short-term, acute care hospital.[7] As for ED visits that resulted in an inpatient admission, an average of 50.2% patients with hepatic encephalopathy had a routine discharge, 22.2% were released to another health institution, 16.2% were transmitted to home health care, and 3.2% were transferred to another hospital.

HOSPITALIZATION BURDEN
Inpatient Admissions

Hepatic encephalopathy is associated with a wide array of neurologic complications that range in severity from changes in psychomotor speed and working memory to more progressive psychiatric manifestations, such as gross disorientation and coma.[5] The developments of major overt neuropsychological symptoms in hepatic encephalopathy has been linked to poor prognosis[9] and substantial health care use and cost burdens.[10] As is the case with cirrhosis-related complications, a large portion of the health care burden of hepatic encephalopathy is related to inpatient hospitalization.[11] Such inpatient burden to the health care system is significant and it has continued to increase during recent years.

In the United States, hepatic encephalopathy accounts for 0.33% of all inpatient admissions.[12] The number of hospital discharges related to hepatic encephalopathy in the United States has increased by 117.7% from 2000 to 2014 (**Fig. 2**). During the same period, the rate of hepatic encephalopathy–related discharges per 100,000 persons increased by 92.7% (9.0 per 100,000 persons in 2000 to 17.4 per 100,000 persons in 2014).[7] Of all hospitalized patients in 2014, 48.8% had a routine discharge and 3.4% were transferred to another short-term hospital, whereas 17.7% were released to home health care. The proportion of patients with hepatic encephalopathy

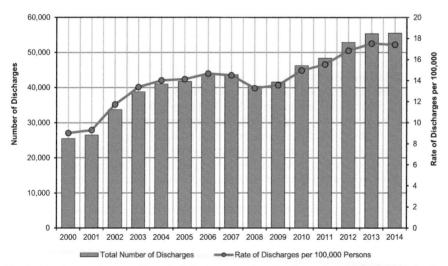

Fig. 2. Number and rates of hospital discharges related to hepatic encephalopathy in the United States, National (Nationwide) Inpatient Sample 2000 to 2014. (Data taken from the HCUPnet, Healthcare Cost and Utilization Project. Agency for Healthcare Research and Quality, Rockville, MD. https://hcupnet.ahrq.gov/.)

who continued to seek treatments at nursing home or rehabilitation facility after discharge has also increased from 18.0% in 2000 to 23.2% in 2014.[7]

Inpatient Length of Stay

The presence of hepatic encephalopathy has been associated with an increase in inpatient length of stay (LOS) among patient with cirrhosis. In a study of the Nationwide Inpatient Sample between 1998 and 2003, patients with hepatic encephalopathy had a 24% longer LOS (95% confidence interval [CI], 22%–26%) compared with cirrhotic patients without hepatic encephalopathy.[13] In similar studies using data from the Nationwide Inpatient Sample, the average inpatient LOS was 8.5 days in 2009 and 8.0 days in 2014.[10,12] Those estimates were comparable to the median LOS of 8 days reported by a data warehouse query study of 316 patients with an incident hepatic encephalopathy hospitalization between April 2010 and February 2012.[14] Significant predictors of longer LOS in hepatic encephalopathy includes the Model for End-Stage Liver Disease score, sex, use of antibiotics (other than rifaximin),[14] elective admission, major of extreme disease severity at admission, weight loss, and the number of procedures performed during hospitalization.[12]

Hospital Readmission

Hepatic cirrhosis is one of the leading causes of hospital readmission in the United States.[15,16] Studies have shown that readmission rates in cirrhosis increase with disease severity and are highest among patients with hepatic decompensations.[17,18] Owing to its recurring nature as a complication of decompensated cirrhosis, hepatic encephalopathy is considered to be a primary risk factor for hospital readmissions among cirrhotic patients.[19–23] Hepatic encephalopathy has also been cited as one of the most common preventable causes of hospital readmission in cirrhosis.[22,24] This is due to the fact that an estimated 60% of qualified patients with hepatic encephalopathy do not receive prophylactic treatments after hospital discharge.[25] Consequently, hepatic encephalopathy is associated with a significant health care burden related to hospital readmissions.[19,26–28]

The association between hepatic encephalopathy and hospital readmissions has been well investigated using survey data from nationally representative samples such as the National Readmission Database and by means of cross-sectional, prospective and retrospective data analyses. In a multicenter, prospective study of 14 cites, 23.7% of enrolled patients with 3-month readmissions had hepatic encephalopathy.[15] Among patients who were readmitted 2 times, 3 times, and 4 or more times within the 3 months after discharge 40.3%, 32.1%, and 61.5% were admitted owing to hepatic encephalopathy, respectively. Results from this study were similar to findings from a multistate population-based cohort study of 119,722 index admissions with cirrhosis where the hepatic encephalopathy–related 30- and 90-day unadjusted readmission rates were 18.1% and 28.8%, respectively.[29] Hepatic encephalopathy was also a significant predictor of both 30- and 90-day hospital readmission in all adjusted models.

In a medical chart review of 140 hepatic encephalopathy admissions between January 1, 2010, and September 30, 2013, one-fourth of patients with hepatic encephalopathy were readmitted during the 90-day interval after the index discharge.[30] Hypertension (62.9% of all enrolled patients) was the sole independent predictor for 90-day readmission adjusted odds ratio (aOR) 4.1 (95% CI, 1.1–14.7). The findings from this study differed from similar studies in that several clinical variables such as diabetes and Model for End-Stage Liver Disease score, which are routinely reported to be independent predictors of readmissions in patients with hepatic encephalopathy,[31] were only associated with an increased odds of readmission in the univariate analyses.[30] The authors suggested that coexisting vascular brain injury related to prolonged elevated blood pressure could explain the association between hypertension and increased admission rates in hepatic encephalopathy.[30,32]

According to a study of 24,473 patients with hepatic encephalopathy from the 2013 National Readmission Database, the 30-day hepatic encephalopathy–related readmission rate was 32.4%.[33] Of all patients with hepatic encephalopathy with readmissions, within 30 days from discharge, 33.9% were due to hepatic encephalopathy. Furthermore, the study found that 40% of patients with hepatic encephalopathy were at a high risk of readmission. Compared with patients with hepatic encephalopathy without a 30-day readmission, those readmitted had a hazard ratio of 4.03 (95% CI, 3.5–4.7) times the risk of calendar-year mortality. Significant predictors of 30-day readmissions included receiving paracentesis, acute kidney injury, and the presence of ascites. The cost of the index hepatic encephalopathy hospitalization was similar between those readmitted and not readmitted ($10,386 vs $10,370; $P = .96$). However, the cost of the first readmission was significantly higher compared with the first admission ($14,198 vs $10,386; $P<.001$).

Shaheen and colleagues[34] used 2014 data from the National Readmission Database to assess readmission rates, costs, and predictors for the 90-day readmissions in patients admitted for cirrhosis or its complications. About one-quarter of the 58,954 cirrhotic index admissions were followed by a 90-day readmission. In 97% of index admissions, 1 or more decompensated cirrhosis states were recorded. The presence of hepatic encephalopathy was more frequent in the readmission group compared with those without readmissions (47% vs 34%; $P<.001$). Hepatic encephalopathy was also associated with 93% higher adjusted odds of 90-day readmissions (aOR, 1.93; 95% CI, 1.85–2.01). Among patients admitted for hepatic encephalopathy during the index admission, having private insurance (aOR, 0.92; 95% CI, 0.84–0.99) and esophageal varices (aOR, 0.55; 95% CI, 0.46–0.66) reduced the odds for the 90-day readmissions, whereas the presence of comorbid ascites increased readmission odds (aOR, 1.19; 95% CI, 1.12–1.28). In 2014, the study found the cost burden of hepatic encephalopathy–related 90-day readmissions to be $0.2 billion.[34]

Cost of Hospitalization

In the United States, the increase in hepatic encephalopathy–related hospitalization rates, translated into an increase of 197.2% in hospital charges between 2000 and 2015 (**Fig. 3**). A study of 1113 patients with hepatic encephalopathy from the 2012 Medicare database found the range of inpatient costs to be between $25,364 and $58,625.[35] The total national inpatient charges related to hepatic encephalopathy in 2014 were $11.9 billion.[10] However, such financial burden does not reflect on the full economic inpatient burden in the United States because 22% of hospitalized patients with hepatic encephalopathy are discharged to other medical institutions (ie, nursing homes or rehabilitation facilities).[7] Factors associated with increased hepatic encephalopathy–related inpatient charges in the United States include the presence of ascites, esophageal varices, hepatorenal syndrome, age, sex, race, major or extreme disease severity at admission, number of procedures, and weight loss.[10,12]

In a study of the economic burden of hepatitis C–associated disease, the mean, minimum, and maximum global costs of hepatic encephalopathy were $9180, $5370, and $50,120, respectively.[36] A retrospective observational study of 7000 inpatients stays related to 5000 patients with hepatic encephalopathy in France found the average cost of hospitalization, from a social security payer perspective, to be €5,535, which translates to €40 million in total annual costs.[37] In this study, an estimated 33%

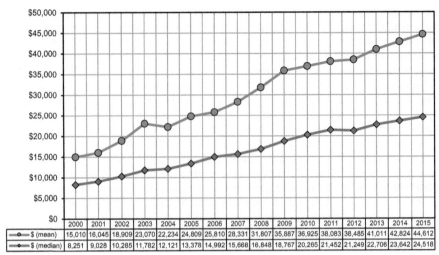

	2000	2001	2002	2003	2004	2005	2006	2007	2008	2009	2010	2011	2012	2013	2014	2015
$ (mean)	15,010	16,045	18,909	23,070	22,234	24,809	25,810	28,331	31,807	35,887	36,925	38,083	38,485	41,011	42,824	44,612
$ (median)	8,251	9,028	10,285	11,782	12,121	13,378	14,992	15,668	16,848	18,767	20,265	21,452	21,249	22,706	23,642	24,518

Fig. 3. Mean and median charges per hospitalization related to hepatic encephalopathy in the United States, National (Nationwide) Inpatient Sample 2000 to 2014. (Data taken from the HCUPnet, Healthcare Cost and Utilization Project. Agency for Healthcare Research and Quality, Rockville, MD. https://hcupnet.ahrq.gov/.)

of the total inpatient cost incurred by patients with a level 4 severity drug-related group. A study of 450 patients with index overt hepatic encephalopathy admission in the Italian Marche region between 2010 and 2012 found the national hospitalization charges of hepatic encephalopathy to be € 200 million in the first year of the index hospitalization.[38]

HEALTH-RELATED QUALITY OF LIFE

The burden of hepatic encephalopathy extends beyond the direct economic aspect of health care use to include costs related to patients' impaired health-related quality of life (HRQOL). Furthermore, hepatic encephalopathy has been associated with significant financial and psychological burdens to caregivers.[39] In a review article of studies published from 1998 to 2018 comparing those with versus those without hepatic encephalopathy, patients with hepatic encephalopathy had poorer HRQOL in 17 of the 21 studies conducted to date.[40] Studies have also shown that history of overt hepatic encephalopathy is associated with long-term impairments to global cognitive function, working memory, and learning.[41,42] Such impairments persisted after liver transplantation.[43]

A prospective study of 118 cirrhosis patients, showed that cognitive reserve was an independent predictor of total sickness impact profile ($P<.001$), psychosocial ($P<.001$), and physical scores ($P<.03$), even after accounting for covert hepatic encephalopathy, Model for End-Stage Liver Disease score, and psychiatric disorders.[44] Similar findings were reported by other investigators.[40] A review article highlighted the impacts of sleep–wake cycle changes on the HRQOL of patients with hepatic encephalopathy.[40] This finding underlines the need to consider cognitive reserve and sleep–wake cycle changes when evaluating patients with cirrhosis and their HRQOL because those with higher cognitive reserve were seen to report better HRQOL.

In addition to poor HRQOL, hepatic encephalopathy has been associated with low socioeconomic status. In a study of 104 patients with cirrhosis, Bajaj and colleagues[45] were the first to examine the socioeconomic and emotional burdens caused by cirrhosis and hepatic encephalopathy to patients and their caregivers. The study found that history of hepatic encephalopathy was correlated with poor performance on almost all the cognition tests, worse employment and economic status. Those findings were confirmed by a multicenter study of 236 patients with cirrhosis, where those with prior overt hepatic encephalopathy episodes fared poorly in almost all cognition tests, fewer were employed in past 12 months (65% vs 18%; $P = .001$), and had lower personal income ($16,000 to $24,999 vs $12,000 to $15,999; $P = .027$), compared with those without prior history of overt hepatic encephalopathy.[46] This finding highlights the need for the implantation of multidisciplinary interventions to address all dimensions (ie, emotional, financial, and socioeconomic) of the substantial burden imposed by hepatic encephalopathy on patients and their caregivers.

PHARMACOECONOMICS OF HEPATIC ENCEPHALOPATHY MANAGEMENT

The primary strategy for managing overt hepatic encephalopathy involves active treatment of any acute episodes of overt hepatic encephalopathy, secondary prophylaxis for recurrence prevention and control of precipitating factors related to overt hepatic encephalopathy manifestation.[5] Guidelines from the American Association for the Study of Liver Disease recommend lactulose as the first choice of overt hepatic encephalopathy treatment. Together, rifaximin is suggested as an add-on treatment to lactulose for the prevention for overt hepatic encephalopathy recurrence. Recommendations for alternative or additional therapies for patients who are nonresponsive to conventional treatments include L-ornithine L-aspartate and branched chain amino acids.[5]

Multiple studies have investigated the impact of treatment options on health care use and economic burdens related to the management of hepatic encephalopathy. Rifaximin and lactulose as a combination therapy has been shown in some studies to decrease both the cost and health care use burdens of hepatic encephalopathy when compared with lactulose alone.[6,47–53] However, most health care use studies conducted to date on the effects of rifaximin plus lactulose combination therapy have several limitations, including small samples size, lack of accounting for confounding by indication, retrospective study designs, and limited use of real-world claims data.

Treatment Options and Inpatient Admissions

The impact of rifaximin on inpatient admissions has been reported using data from both observational and experimental study designs. Although some studies have shown lower hospitalization rates for those treated with rifaximin, similar results were not found in other studies. In a multicenter observational study of 145 hepatic encephalopathy patient in the United Kingdom, inpatient resource use was compared in 6 months before versus the 6 months after rifaximin-α initiation.[48] Compared with the 6 months before initiations, rifaximin-α was associated with a significant reduction in the number of both liver-related (from 1.3 to 0.5; $P<.001$) and all-cause–related (from 1.9 to 0.9; $P<.001$) inpatient admissions. Rifaximin-α initiation was also shown to significantly decrease the number of ED visits in the 6 months but not in the 12 months after initiation.[48] In a double-blind randomized controlled trial, rifaximin was associated with a 9% lower rate of hepatic encephalopathy–related hospitalization compared with placebo.[54] In a 24-month open-label maintenance trial, long-term exposure to rifaximin (550 mg, twice daily) was associated with a decrease in both all-cause and hepatic encephalopathy–related hospitalization rates.[55]

In contrast, a study of 82 patients who crossed over from the placebo arm of 6 months rifaximin versus a placebo-controlled trial into a 24-month open-label main-tenance study found no significant difference in hepatic encephalopathy–related hos-pitalizations during the rifaximin versus placebo treatment periods.[56] In a multicenter prospective observational study of 265 patients who experienced at least 1 overt he-patic encephalopathy episode, within 30 days before enrollment, 23 patients, of whom 21 were on rifaximin, accounted for 73 (60%) of all observed hepatic encephalopathy occurrences. An estimated 88% of all observed 73 hepatic encephalopathy episodes resulted in hospital admissions.[57] A retrospective study of 606 patients with hepatic encephalopathy using United States pharmacy claims data found no significant differ-ence in hepatic encephalopathy–related hospitalization rates for rifaximin plus lactu-lose (16.0%) versus lactulose monotherapy (15.3%) (P = .841).[58]

Treatment Options and Inpatient Length of Stay

Studies have shown that treatment with rifaximin alone or in combination with lactu-lose is associated with reductions in the length of hospital stays for patients with he-patic encephalopathy. In a multicenter study of 145 hepatic encephalopathy patient in the United Kingdom, all-cause and liver-related hospital bed days were reduced by 62% and 58% after rifaximin-α initiation, respectively.[48] Another observational study of 326 patients with hepatic encephalopathy in the United Kingdom found treatment with rifaximin to be associated with decreases in inpatient LOS by 31% to 53% when compared with the period before rifaximin commencement.[59] In a prospective double-blind randomized study, patients on rifaximin plus lactulose had shorter hos-pital stays compared with those on lactulose plus placebo (5.8 days vs 8.2 days; P = .001).[60] A small retrospective study of 39 patients with hepatic encephalopathy with end-stage liver disease reported shorter LOS for those on rifaximin versus lactu-lose (3.5 days vs 5.0 days; P<.0001).[61] Leevy and Phillips[62] reported similar results in a study of 145 patients with hepatic encephalopathy where those on rifaximin had 4.8 fewer days hospitalized than those on lactulose alone.

Treatment Options Hospital Readmission

Studies on the effects of rifaximin monotherapy and in combination with lactulose on reductions in hospital readmissions have been inconclusive. Namely, rifaximin-α use was correlated with lower 30 days inpatient readmissions from both all-causes (before use vs after use 0.5 vs 0.2; P = .039) and liver-related (before use vs after use 0.5 vs 0.2; P = .039) at 6 months of follow-up.[48] However, the effect of rifaximin-α intuition on the number of 30 days inpatient readmissions was not significant at 12 months from follow-up. In contrast, a retrospective study of 178 patients with hepatic encephalop-athy in the United States found no significant difference in the 30-day hospitalization readmissions for rifaximin plus lactulose versus lactulose alone (30 days 11.7% vs 7.1%, respectively; P = .527).[63] However, in this study, significantly lower hepatic encephalopathy–related hospital readmissions for rifaximin plus lactulose versus lac-tulose were only observed in the 180-day observation period (16.2% vs 2.4%, respec-tively; P = .028).

Treatment Options and Economic Burden of Hepatic Encephalopathy

Few studies have investigated the difference in crude hepatic encephalopathy–related health care charges between rifaximin plus lactulose versus lactulose alone. In the ma-jority of the research published to date, rifaximin plus lactulose has been shown to decrease health care cost owing to the decrease in hospitalization rates after hepatic encephalopathy; however, the evidence remains inconclusive. A medical chart review of 39 patients with hepatic encephalopathy conducted by Neff and colleagues[61] reported lower cost of therapy per patient for those who were on lactulose plus rifaximin (15 patients) compared with those on just lactulose (24 patients) ($13,285 vs $7958). In another chart review study of 145 patients with hepatic encephalopathy, hospitalization charges per patient were $14,222 and $56,635 for those on lactulose plus rifaximin and lactulose alone, respectively.[62] However, both studies reported a crude difference in health care charges and neither provided any measures of statistical significance.

Rifaximin plus lactulose was shown in another study to results in lower but statistically insignificant per patient average health care cost when compared with lactulose monotherapy ($50,542 vs $61,545, respectively; $P = .055$).[64] An Italian economic analysis found rifaximin 550 mg twice daily to decrease the net cost per patient owing to decrease in hepatic encephalopathy recurrences leading to hospitalizations.[53] A cost analysis of rifaximin use in the United Kingdom found reduction from £12,522 to £5915 in annual inpatient expenditures before versus after treatment commencement, respectively.[59] Such expenditure reduction equated to £3228 of annual savings per patient even after accounting for the cost of a 1-year supply of rifaximin (£3379).[59]

The cost effectiveness of rifaximin plus lactulose in comparison to lactulose monotherapy has been examined in multiple studies. A cost-effectiveness decision analysis of 6 hepatic encephalopathy treatment strategies found rifaximin monotherapy not to be cost effective at the reported drug wholesale prices.[65] However, Huang and colleagues[65] found rifaximin salvage therapy for lactulose-refractory patients to be cost effective. Several European based studies quantified the incremental cost-effectiveness ratios of rifaximin in combination with lactulose versus lactulose alone in patients with recurrent hepatic encephalopathy.[6] In France, Kabeshova and colleagues[66] found the 2- and 5-year incremental cost-effectiveness ratios for rifaximin plus lactulose versus lactulose alone to be €19,187 and €18,517 per quality-adjusted life-year, respectively. Similar results were reported in Belgian, Dutch, and Swedish studies, where the 5-year incremental cost-effectiveness ratios of rifaximin plus lactulose versus lactulose alone were €21,547, €9576, and €17,918, respectively.[6,67–69]

SUMMARY

Owing to its recurring nature as a neuropsychiatric complication of decompensated cirrhosis, hepatic encephalopathy poses substantial economic and use burdens to the health care system. Such health care burden is significant, and it continued to increase during recent years. In the United States, hepatic encephalopathy accounts for 0.33% of all inpatient admissions. The number of hospital discharges related to hepatic encephalopathy has increased by 117.7% from 2000 to 2014. The increase in hepatic encephalopathy–related hospitalization rates translated into an increase of 197.2% in hospital charges between 2000 and 2015. The presence of hepatic encephalopathy has also been associated with longer inpatient LOS and high risk of hospital readmissions among patient with cirrhosis. The effects of hepatic encephalopathy extends beyond the direct economic and use burdens to include costs related to patients' impaired HRQOL. Rifaximin plus lactulose, as a combination therapy for hepatic encephalopathy, has been shown in some studies to decrease both the cost and health care use burdens of hepatic encephalopathy when compared with lactulose alone. However, most health care use studies conducted to date on the effects of this combination therapy have several limitations.

DISCLOSURE

The authors in this article have no relevant financial or other relationships to disclose.

REFERENCES

1. Asrani SK, Devarbhavi H, Eaton J, et al. Burden of liver diseases in the world. J Hepatol 2019;70(1):151–71.
2. Marcellin P, Kutala BK. Liver diseases: a major, neglected global public health problem requiring urgent actions and large-scale screening. Liver Int 2018; 38(Suppl 1):2–6.
3. Allen AM, Van Houten HK, Sangaralingham LR, et al. Healthcare cost and utilization in nonalcoholic fatty liver disease: real-world data from a large U.S. claims database. Hepatology 2018;68(6):2230–8.
4. Mellinger JL, Shedden K, Winder GS, et al. The high burden of alcoholic cirrhosis in privately insured persons in the United States. Hepatology 2018;68(3):872–82.
5. Vilstrup H, Amodio P, Bajaj J, et al. Hepatic encephalopathy in chronic liver disease: 2014 Practice Guideline by the American Association for the Study of Liver Diseases and the European Association for the Study of the Liver. Hepatology 2014;60(2):715–35.
6. Neff G, Zachry W III. Systematic review of the economic burden of overt hepatic encephalopathy and pharmacoeconomic impact of rifaximin. Pharmacoeconomics 2018;36:809–22.
7. HCUPnet. Emergency Department National Statistics. Healthcare cost and utilization project agency for healthcare research and quality. Rockville (MD): U.S. Department of Health & Human Services; 2019. Available at: https://hcupnet. ahrq.gov/. Accessed April 26, 2019.
8. Sarvepalli S, Garg SK, Singh D, et al. Utilization of emergency department for hepatic encephalopathy: examination of national trends (2006-2014). Paper presented at: Hepatology. San Francisco, November 9 - 13, 2018.
9. Wong RJ, Gish RG, Ahmed A. Hepatic encephalopathy is associated with significantly increased mortality among patients awaiting liver transplantation. Liver Transpl 2014;20(12):1454–61.
10. Hirode G, Vittinghoff E, Wong RJ. Increasing burden of hepatic encephalopathy among hospitalized adults: an analysis of the 2010-2014 National Inpatient Sample. Dig Dis Sci 2019;64(6):1448–57.
11. Patidar KR, Thacker LR, Wade JB, et al. Covert hepatic encephalopathy is independently associated with poor survival and increased risk of hospitalization. Am J Gastroenterol 2014;109:1757–63.
12. Stepanova M, Mishra A, Venkatesan C, et al. In-hospital mortality and economic burden associated with hepatic encephalopathy in the United States from 2005 to 2009. Clin Gastroenterol Hepatol 2012;10:1034–41.e1.
13. Nguyen GC, Segev DL, Thuluvath PJ. Nationwide increase in hospitalizations and hepatitis C among inpatients with cirrhosis and sequelae of portal hypertension. Clin Gastroenterol Hepatol 2007;5:1092–9.
14. Martel-Laferrière V, Homberger C, Bichoupan K, et al. MELD score and antibiotics use are predictors of length of stay in patients hospitalized with hepatic encephalopathy. BMC Gastroenterol 2014;14:1–6.
15. Bajaj JS, Reddy KR, Tandon P, et al. The 3-month readmission rate remains unacceptably high in a large North American cohort of patients with cirrhosis. Hepatology 2016;64:200–8.

16. Fontanarosa PB, McNutt RA. Revisiting hospital readmissions. JAMA 2013; 309(4):398–400.
17. Berman K, Tandra S, Forssell K, et al. Incidence and predictors of 30-day readmission among patients hospitalized for advanced liver disease. Clin Gastroenterol Hepatol 2011;9(3):254–9.
18. Fagan KJ, Zhao EY, Horsfall LU, et al. Burden of decompensated cirrhosis and ascites on hospital services in a tertiary care facility: time for change? Intern Med J 2014;44:865–72.
19. Orman ES, Ghabril M, Emmett TW, et al. Hospital readmissions in patients with cirrhosis: a systematic review. J Hosp Med 2018;13:490–5.
20. Tapper EB, Finkelstein D, Mittleman MA, et al. A quality improvement initiative reduces 30-day rate of readmission for patients with cirrhosis. Clin Gastroenterol Hepatol 2016;14(5):753–9.
21. Seraj SM, Campbell EJ, Argyropoulos SK, et al. Hospital readmissions in decompensated cirrhotics: factors pointing toward a prevention strategy. World J Gastroenterol 2017;23:6868–76.
22. Scaglione SJ, Metcalfe L, Kliethermes S, et al. Early hospital readmissions and mortality in patients with decompensated cirrhosis enrolled in a large national health insurance administrative database. J Clin Gastroenterol 2017;51:839–44.
23. Okafor PN, Nnadi AK, Okoli O, et al. Same- vs different-hospital readmissions in patients with cirrhosis after hospital discharge. Am J Gastroenterol 2019;114: 464–71.
24. Volk ML, Tocco RS, Bazick J, et al. Hospital readmissions among patients with decompensated cirrhosis. Am J Gastroenterol 2012;107(2):247.
25. Neff G, Frederick T. Assessing treatment patterns in patients with overt hepatic encephalopathy: 1612. Paper presented in the 2012 Liver Meeting. Boston, November 9-13, 2012.
26. Saab S. Evaluation of the impact of rehospitalization in the management of hepatic encephalopathy. Int J Gen Med 2015;8:165.
27. Suraweera D, Sundaram V, Saab S. Evaluation and management of hepatic encephalopathy: current status and future directions. Gut Liver 2016;10:509–19.
28. Ge PS, Runyon BA. Treatment of patients with cirrhosis. N Engl J Med 2016; 375(8):767–77.
29. Tapper EB, Halbert B, Mellinger J. Rates of and reasons for hospital readmissions in patients with cirrhosis: a multistate population-based cohort study. Clin Gastroenterol Hepatol 2016;14(8):1181–8.e2.
30. Rassameehiran S, Mankongpaisarnrung C, Sutamtewagul G, et al. Predictor of 90-day readmission rate for hepatic encephalopathy. South Med J 2016;109: 365–9.
31. Desai AP, Reau N. The burden of rehospitalization for patients with liver cirrhosis. Hosp Pract (1995) 2016;44:60–9.
32. Maillard P, Seshadri S, Beiser A, et al. Effects of systolic blood pressure on white-matter integrity in young adults in the Framingham Heart Study: a cross-sectional study. Lancet Neurol 2012;11(12):1039–47.
33. Kruger AJ, Aberra F, Black SM, et al. A validated risk model for prediction of early readmission in patients with hepatic encephalopathy. Ann Hepatol 2019;18: 310–7.
34. Shaheen AA, Nguyen HH, Congly SE, et al. Nationwide estimates and risk factors of hospital readmission in patients with cirrhosis in the United States. Liver Int 2019;39:878–84.

35. Irish W, Saynisch P, Mallow PJ, et al. Using the Medicare claims database to understand the economic burden of liver disease: a case study in hepatic encephalopathy. Value Health 2015;18(3):A226.
36. El Khoury AC, Wallace C, Klimack WK, et al. Economic burden of hepatitis C-associated diseases: Europe, Asia Pacific, and the Americas. J Med Econ 2012;15:887–96.
37. Amaz C, Blein C, Benamouzig R, et al. Economic burden of hospitalization for hepatic encephalopathy in France: an analysis of cost discriminating factors by patient profile. Value in Health 2016;19(7):A511.
38. Sciattella P, Mennini FS, Marcellusi A, et al. Clinical outcomes and hospital costs of hepatic encephalopathy: an analysis of "real life" data from Marche Region. Recent Prog Med 2018;109:585–94.
39. Montagnese S, Amato E, Schiff S, et al. A patients' and caregivers' perspective on hepatic encephalopathy. Metab Brain Dis 2012;27:567–72.
40. Montagnese S, Bajaj JS. Impact of hepatic encephalopathy in cirrhosis on quality-of-life issues. Drugs 2019;79:11–6.
41. Bajaj JS, Schubert CM, Heuman DM, et al. Persistence of cognitive impairment after resolution of overt hepatic encephalopathy. Gastroenterology 2010;138(7): 2332–40.
42. Umapathy S, Dhiman RK, Grover S, et al. Persistence of cognitive impairment after resolution of overt hepatic encephalopathy. Am J Gastroenterol 2014; 109(7):1011.
43. Campagna F, Montagnese S, Schiff S, et al. Cognitive impairment and electroencephalographic alterations before and after liver transplantation: what is reversible? Liver Transpl 2014;20(8):977–86.
44. Patel AV, Wade JB, Thacker LR, et al. Cognitive reserve is a determinant of health-related quality of life in patients with cirrhosis, independent of covert hepatic encephalopathy and model for end-stage liver disease score. Clin Gastroenterol Hepatol 2015;13:987–91.
45. Bajaj JS, Wade JB, Gibson DP, et al. The multi-dimensional burden of cirrhosis and hepatic encephalopathy on patients and caregivers. Am J Gastroenterol 2011;106:1646–53.
46. Bajaj JS, Riggio O, Allampati S, et al. Cognitive dysfunction is associated with poor socioeconomic status in patients with cirrhosis: an international multicenter study. Clin Gastroenterol Hepatol 2013;11:1511–6.
47. Flamm SL. Considerations for the cost-effective management of hepatic encephalopathy. Am J Manag Care 2018;24:S51–61.
48. Hudson M, Radwan A, Di Maggio P, et al. The impact of rifaximin-α on the hospital resource use associated with the management of patients with hepatic encephalopathy: a retrospective observational study (IMPRESS). Frontline Gastroenterol 2017;8:243–51.
49. Krag A, Schuchmann M, Sodatonou H, et al. Design of the prospective real-world outcomes study of hepatic encephalopathy Patients' Experience on Rifaximin-alpha (PROSPER): an observational study among 550 patients. Hepatol Med Policy 2018;3:4.
50. Leevy CB. Economic impact of treatment options for hepatic encephalopathy. Semin Liver Dis 2007;27:26–31.
51. Neff G. Pharmacoeconomics of hepatic encephalopathy. Pharmacotherapy 2010;30:28s–32s.
52. Patel D, McPhail MJ, Cobbold JF, et al. Hepatic encephalopathy. Br J Hosp Med (Lond) 2012;73:79–85.

53. Roggeri DP, Roggeri A. Economic impact of the use of rifaximin 550 mg twice daily for the treatment of overt hepatic encephalopathy in Italy. Hepat Med 2017;9:37–43.
54. Bass NM, Mullen KD, Sanyal A, et al. Rifaximin treatment in hepatic encephalopathy. N Engl J Med 2010;362(12):1071–81.
55. Mullen KD, Sanyal AJ, Bass NM, et al. Rifaximin is safe and well tolerated for long-term maintenance of remission from overt hepatic encephalopathy. Clin Gastroenterol Hepatol 2014;12:1390–7.e2.
56. Bajaj JS, Barrett AC, Bortey E, et al. Prolonged remission from hepatic encephalopathy with rifaximin: results of a placebo crossover analysis. Aliment Pharmacol Ther 2015;41:39–45.
57. Landis CS, Ghabril M, Rustgi V, et al. Prospective multicenter observational study of overt hepatic encephalopathy. Dig Dis Sci 2016;61:1728–34.
58. Hammond D, Dayama N, Martin B. Impact of rifaximin and lactulose versus lactulose alone on hospitalization for acute recurrent hepatic encephalopathy. Paper presented at: Value in Health. New York: Elsevier Science Inc; 2017.
59. Orr JG, Currie CJ, Berni E, et al. The impact on hospital resource utilisation of treatment of hepatic encephalopathy with rifaximin-alpha. Liver Int 2016;36: 1295–303.
60. Sharma BC, Sharma P, Lunia MK, et al. A randomized, double-blind, controlled trial comparing rifaximin plus lactulose with lactulose alone in treatment of overt hepatic encephalopathy. Am J Gastroenterol 2013;108(9):1458.
61. Neff G, Kemmer N, Zacharias V, et al. Analysis of hospitalizations comparing rifaximin versus lactulose in the management of hepatic encephalopathy. Transplantation proceedings. Elsevier; 2006. p. 3552-5.
62. Leevy CB, Phillips JA. Hospitalizations during the use of rifaximin versus lactulose for the treatment of hepatic encephalopathy. Dig Dis Sci 2007;52(3):737–41.
63. Courson A, Jones GM, Twilla JD. Treatment of acute hepatic encephalopathy: comparing the effects of adding rifaximin to lactulose on patient outcomes. J Pharm Pract 2016;29(3):212–7.
64. Neff GW, Kemmer N, Duncan C, et al. Update on the management of cirrhosis - focus on cost-effective preventative strategies. Clinicoecon Outcomes Res 2013; 5:143–52.
65. Huang E, Esrailian E, Spiegel B. The cost-effectiveness and budget impact of competing therapies in hepatic encephalopathy–a decision analysis. Aliment Pharmacol Ther 2007;26(8):1147–61.
66. Kabeshova A, Ben Hariz S, Tsakeu E, et al. Cost-effectiveness analysis of rifaximin-α administration for the reduction of episodes of overt hepatic encephalopathy in recurrence compared with standard treatment in France. Therap Adv Gastroenterol 2016;9(4):473–82.
67. Whitehouse J, Berni E, Conway P, et al. Evaluation of the cost effectiveness and societal impact of rifaximin-A 550mg in the reduction of recurrence of overt hepatic encephalopathy in The Netherlands. Value in Health 2015;18(7):A629.
68. Poole C, Berni E, Conway P, et al. Evaluation of the cost effectiveness of Rifaximin-á 550mg in the reduction of recurrence of overt hepatic encephalopathy in Sweden. Value in Health 2015;18(7):A626.
69. Berni E, Connolly M, Conway P, et al. Evaluation of the cost effectiveness of Rifaximin-Á in the reduction of recurrence of overt hepatic encephalopathy in Belgium. Value in Health 2015;18(7):A628.

Long-Term Management
Modern Measures to Prevent Readmission in Patients with Hepatic Encephalopathy

Russell Rosenblatt, MD, Johnathan Yeh, PA, Paul J. Gaglio, MD*

KEYWORDS

- Hepatic encephalopathy • Wearable technology • Telemedicine • Apps
- Automated medication dispensers • Text message alerts

KEY POINTS

- Prevention of initial hospitalizations as well as readmissions in patients with hepatic encephalopathy (HE) will require a multidisciplinary approach including patient and family education regarding the signs and symptoms of HE.
- Home-based patient self-assessment tools to recognize and treat HE may be valuable.
- Improved medication adherence can be achieved using text alerts, phone apps, as well as home-based automated medicine-dispensing platforms.
- Telemedicine, including remote telemonitoring, patient and family tele-education, on-demand teleconsultation, and virtual patient-clinician visits, may diminish HE progression and hospital admissions.
- Wearable technology has the future potential to monitor multiple aspects of HE, including asterixis, falls, changes in electroencephalogram, and serum ammonia levels, and may allow early recognition and treatment of HE to prevent hospitalization and readmissions.

INTRODUCTION

Hepatic encephalopathy (HE) is a frequent, costly, morbid complication of cirrhosis. Beginning with the demonstration of a relationship between neomycin and a decrease in serum ammonia levels in 1957, various medical therapies have been used to improve outcomes in patients with HE.[1] Lactulose[2] combined with rifaximin,[3] a more recently approved nonabsorbable antibiotic, are currently the mainstays of medical therapy and have proven benefit to prevent both recurrence and hospitalizations for HE. Novel therapeutics targeting different pathobiological mechanisms that induce HE, such as fecal microbiota transplant,[4] offer the potential for improved patient outcomes.

Department of Medicine, Center for Liver Disease and Transplantation, NY-Presbyterian Hospital, Columbia University Medical Center, Columbia University College of Physicians and Surgeons, PH-14 622 West 168th Street, New York, NY 10032, USA
* Corresponding author.
E-mail address: pg2011@cumc.columbia.edu

Clin Liver Dis 24 (2020) 277–290
https://doi.org/10.1016/j.cld.2020.01.007
1089-3261/20/© 2020 Elsevier Inc. All rights reserved.

Despite multiple treatment options, HE is a frequent indication for hospitalization and represents a common manifestation of portal hypertension and decompensated liver disease that contributes to hospital readmissions.[5–7] Thus, HE represents a major health care challenge to patients, physicians, and hospital systems; multiple new techniques are being evaluated to assist in preventing readmissions in these high-risk patients. These different approaches include providing easier access to medications; the ability to self-diagnose and initiate therapy for HE; and advances in technology such as automated medication dispensing, reminders to take medication via text messaging, telemedicine, and, perhaps most importantly, providing home and point-of-care engagement of the patient and family to prevent HE progression and prevent readmissions. This article discusses current and potential future techniques to improve outcomes in these vulnerable patients.

HOSPITALIZATION, READMISSIONS, AND COSTS

Overt HE is present in 10% to 14% of patients at the time of diagnosis of cirrhosis, and it is expected that, in their lifetimes, nearly 30% to 40% of patients with cirrhosis experience overt HE.[8] Hospitalizations for patients with cirrhosis and HE are therefore common, are increasing,[9] and portend a poor prognosis. A recent analysis of a national database revealed that HE was the indication for admission in 0.33% of hospitalizations overall but was associated with a mortality of greater than 15%.[10] An additional study that followed more than 100 patients with cirrhosis who developed their first episode of acute HE indicated that only 42% survived 1 year.[11]

However, for patients hospitalized with cirrhosis, frequent readmissions are equally problematic. Volk and colleagues[12] identified a 37% 1-month readmission rate in patients with decompensated cirrhosis. In a multistate cohort, Tapper and colleagues[5] showed a 12% 30-day readmission rate in cirrhotic patients but identified HE as the most common indication for readmission. A systematic review showed that nearly 40% of patients who were admitted for HE were readmitted within 1 year.[13] It is also apparent that hospitalization rates for HE may vary when comparing academic with community hospitals, where most individuals receive their care. A recently published analysis of hospital admissions in the Mayo Clinic Health System showed that HE-related readmissions were 3 times more common in community hospitals compared with the academic centers.[14] Although the causes for HE readmissions vary and may be related to progression of cirrhosis and portal hypertension, several studies have shown that nonadherence to lactulose was the most common precipitant of hospital readmission for HE.[15,16]

Regrettably, as hospitalizations for HE become increasingly common, costs remain problematic and seem to be increasing.[10,14] A recently published meta-analysis of 16 studies noted that overall costs associated with HE vary, ranging from $5,370 to $50,120.[17] In addition, both indirect and direct costs related to hospitalizations for HE are significant, ranging from $25,364 to $58,625.[17] In total, it is estimated that the annual costs associated with HE in 2009 were as high as $2 billion in the United States.[10]

An additional burden related to managing HE is the cost of medical therapy and the ability to access HE therapy. It is clear that lactulose and rifaximin combination therapy are valuable to prevent and treat HE[3,18] and are cost-effective[3,17,19–21]; however, the monthly cost of rifaximin may be 10-fold higher than that of lactulose. Therefore, techniques to improve access to HE therapy are paramount.

Accessing Hepatic Encephalopathy Therapy

Several recently published studies note that adherence to HE therapy is problematic for many patients; data available from 2011 indicate that more than 60% of patients are not discharged on any HE medications after a hospitalization for HE or do not fill their prescriptions for HE medications,[22] only 54% of patients are adherent to lactulose after an initial episode of overt HE,[16] and 3 in 10 patients have problems affording HE therapy, particularly rifaximin.[23] Anecdotal evidence from our transplant program reveals that, in patients with inadequate insurance and prescription coverage, the out-of-pocket copay for rifaximin can range from $200 to more than $1000 per month. An additional concern in patients with Medicare-based and Medicaid-based insurance is difficulty achieving year-round access to medication when entering the so-called donut hole or coverage gap, described as follows: patients with basic Medicare part D coverage pay 100% of their drug costs until they reach a defined deductible amount (in 2019, this amount is $415). After reaching this deductible, patients pay 25% of the cost of their drugs, and the part D plan pays the rest, until the total spent by the patient and the plan reaches $3820. Once this donut hole is reached, the patient is now responsible for the full cost of all drugs until the total reaches the yearly out-of-pocket spending limit of $4550 as of 2019. Therefore, in patients who enter the donut hole, the patient's out-of-pocket cost for medication may be nearly $1000. However, patients who are in the donut hole may be ineligible for pharmaceutical company assistance programs. Based on these difficulties accessing therapy for HE, several options may be pursued to enhance access to medications.

Manufacturer's Coupons

Given the overall expense of rifaximin, which may contribute to difficulty in accessing and adhering to therapy, multiple different options exist. One example is the availability of a coupon program for non–government-insured patients provided by the manufacture of rifaximin (Xifaxin), which can reduce a patient's copay to less than $100 per month. This cost may be decreased further with additional coupons. However, this program is not accessible to patients covered by government-managed insurance plans such as Medicare and Medicaid.

Charity Care and Specialty Pharmacies

Other alternative options to allow access to HE medication include the use of charity care or specialty pharmacies. One example of charity care is the Patient Access Network (https://panfoundation.org/index.php/en/), which relies on donations from individuals and corporations to assist patients in obtaining access to medical therapies. An additional resource to improve patient access to HE medication includes specialty pharmacies. In offices without dedicated staff to assist in helping patients achieve access to medications, including filling out prior authorization forms and speaking with insurance company representatives, specialty pharmacies can be invaluable. Many specialty pharmacies have expertise in obtaining insurance approvals and are effective in providing access to medications such as rifaximin, immunosuppression, and hepatitis medications.

PATIENT-ASSOCIATED AND FAMILY-ASSOCIATED TECHNIQUES TO PREVENT READMISSION
Recognition of Signs/Symptoms of Hepatic Encephalopathy

As described earlier, both hospitalizations and readmissions in patients with HE are common. It is therefore intuitive that methodologies for patients or their family members to recognize HE and identify when HE is progressing from covert to overt would be valuable, because therapy could be initiated when HE is recognized or progresses. Such methodologies would allow the patient's health care providers to be notified and provide advice regarding therapy to prevent progression of HE and potentially avoid hospital admissions. Potential applications of technology that may be valuable in this regard are summarized next.

Family or Patient Recognition of Signs and Symptoms of Hepatic Encephalopathy

There are multiple signs and symptoms of HE that patients and their families can be taught to recognize, allowing early intervention by the patient's health care provider. Cognitive findings in patients with minimal or covert HE (CHE) may be subtle, and may be difficult to diagnose by health care providers without using specialized testing. However, family members with knowledge and experience related to the patient's baseline personality are often highly attuned to the subtle changes that occur in early HE and CHE and are, in our experience, often able to recognize these changes more effectively than the patient's health care team. In contradistinction, the more overt findings of HE, such as impairment in attention, reaction time, and memory, can be easily recognized by family members, prompting a call to the patient's health care provider and allowing early intervention. In addition, easily recognizable disturbances in the diurnal sleep pattern (sleeping during the day, awake at night) are common initial manifestations of HE that can be readily identified by patients' families. As HE progresses even further, patients may develop mood changes (euphoria or depression), disorientation, inappropriate behavior, somnolence, and confusion, all additional signs that family members can be taught to recognize.

In addition to signs and symptoms, there are several easily recognized physical examination findings in HE. Neuromuscular impairment in patients with overt HE includes bradykinesia, asterixis (flapping motions of outstretched, dorsiflexed hands), slurred speech, and ataxia. In our practice, we have taught patients and their family members how to recognize HE by demonstrating the physical examination finding of asterixis and instructing the family to give an extra dose of lactulose and call us when asterixis is present. Anecdotal evidence from our liver transplant program indicates that multiple hospital admissions have been prevented using this technique.

Patient-Directed and Family-Directed Assessment Tools to Diagnose and Monitor Hepatic Encephalopathy

There are several pencil-and-paper and computerized tests that have been developed for the psychometric evaluation of patients with HE, including the psychometric hepatic encephalopathy score (PHES), line tracing test (LTT), serial dotting test (SDT), digit symbol test (DST), number connection test, repeatable battery for the assessment of neuropsychological status (RBANS), the inhibitory control test (ICT), and the cognitive drug research battery (reviewed in Ref.[24]).

These tests need to be administered and interpreted by a trained health care provider. However, several simple applications, including smartphone, computer, and other assessment tools, have recently been developed that are validated to diagnose CHE or minimal HE and identify this condition to allow therapy to prevent progression to overt HE. These tests are easy to administer and could potentially be performed by the patients and interpreted by the patients' families. The advantage of these tests are that no medical or research training is required to administer them. Examples include the Stroop smartphone application (EncephalApp_Stroop) as published by Bajaj and colleagues,[25] an easily administered test using a smartphone app that has been identified as a valid, reliable tool to screen for CHE or minimal HE.[26] The Stroop test assesses psychomotor speed and cognitive flexibility and thus evaluates the functioning of the anterior attention system, which is impaired in patients with CHE. Specifically, there are 2 stimuli that are assessed: neutral or congruent stimuli whereby the patient is asked to identify the color of a symbol, and incongruent stimuli whereby, as an example, the word red is in the color green, and the patient is asked to identify the color of the word. A total time to complete the Stroop test of greater than 190 seconds identified all patients with CHE with an area under the receiver operator characteristic value of 0.91. In addition, the area under the receiver operator characteristic value was 0.88 for the diagnosis of CHE in those without overt HE. The investigators also noted that test and retest reliability was high among 30 patients retested 1 to 3 months apart. The EncephalApp_Stroop is available on iTunes for free download (http://encephalapp.com/) and a Stroop test for android phones is also available (https://apkpure.com/stroop-color/com.tekxudus.stroop).

Animal naming test
Several recent publications have described the animal naming test (ANT) as a technique to diagnose minimal HE. The ANT determines the maximum number of animals that can be named in 1 minute. In 1 study, 40 control patients with inflammatory bowel disease and 327 consecutive patients with cirrhosis underwent assessment via the ANT.[27] These results were correlated with psychometric HE score and electroencephalography. It was determined after adjusting for age and education that a simplified ANT score of less than 10 animals in 60 seconds was abnormal and the inability to name 15 animals produced the best discrimination between unimpaired patients and those with minimal HE. The ANT has been validated by other investigators as a valuable way to screen for CHE.[28] Additional investigations regarding the validity of these point-of-care diagnostic tests have been performed. In a recent publication, Tapper and colleagues[29] identified several published studies that used at-home or point-of-care testing for HE, including ICT, EncephalApp Stroop, and the ANT. Although the investigators noted that data comparing the performance of each modality are lacking and longitudinal data are limited, there was a suggestion that good performance on the ICT, EncephalApp, or ANT is associated with reduced risk of developing overt HE. **Table 1** lists several tools that may be used to assess cognitive defects in HE.

The obvious advantages of patient-directed and family-directed self-assessment tools for HE, including the EncephalApp and ANT, are the ability to administer these tests at home and on demand to monitor for the presence of either covert or overt HE or when there is concern about the presence of these manifestations of HE. The disadvantages of these tools include the potential for inaccuracy related to result interpretation by the patient or family member caused by either limited education or technologic ability, and patient improvement in performance on the tests with repetition, thus diminishing the ability to correctly identify future HE events.

OTHER TECHNOLOGIES TO PREVENT READMISSION AND ENHANCE MEDICATION ADHERENCE

In general, long-term adherence to medications required to manage chronic disease is poor. Related to HE, the adverse effects of lactulose diminish long-term medication compliance in many patients, because aversion to the taste, and the development of diarrhea, bloating, excessive flatulence, dehydration, hypokalemia, hyponatremia, and other electrolyte disturbances, may be limiting. Lactulose dosing frequency and volume may be diminished in patients taking rifaximin; however, the patients need to adhere to their rifaximin dosing schedules. Therefore, techniques to enhance medication adherence are of utmost importance in patients with HE. Because increased numbers of patients and their families have access to technology, including smartphones, computers, and wearable technologies, these modalities have potential broad applicability in both diagnosing HE as well as preventing progression.

Table 1
Assessment tools for hepatic encephalopathy

Method	Advantage	Disadvantage
Signs/symptoms of HE	Simple to teach Can initiate therapy when recognized	Need family members to be trained May not work if family members are not present
PHES	Validated for HE	Needs to be administered by health care provider
LTT	Validated for HE	Needs to be administered by health care provider
SDT	Validated for HE	Needs to be administered by health care provider
DST	Validated for HE	Needs to be administered by health care provider
Number connection test	Validated for HE	Needs to be administered by health care provider
RBANS	Validated for HE	Needs to be administered by health care provider
ICT	Validated for HE	Needs to be administered by health care provider
Stroop test	Validated for HE Can be performed on demand in patient's home	Need access to the app and ability to use it Possible difficulty interpreting results
ANT	Validated for HE Can be performed on demand in patient's home	Improvement in performance with repetition; possible inaccuracy for future testing

Text Alerts to Remind Patients to Take Medications

It is clear that poor adherence to medications has several severe consequences, including requirement for initial or recurrent hospitalization, increased need for medical interventions, as well as increased morbidity and mortality. In addition, medication nonadherence can result in dramatically increased health care costs, with estimates from North America of approximately $100 billion spent annually and $2000 spent per patient per year in excess physician visits.[30] It is therefore apparent that convenient, wide-reaching techniques are required to enhance medication adherence. Recent technological innovations, including the use of mobile digital devices, apps, smartphones, tablet computers, or personal digital assistants, have been developed; this technology has value as a technique to improve patient health via appointment reminders as well as prompts to take medications. A recently published meta-analysis regarding the use of personalized daily text messaging to enhance medication adherence revealed that text messaging significantly improved medication adherence (odds ratio, 2.11; 95% confidence interval, 1.52–2.93; $P<.001$), approximately doubling the odds of medication adherence compared with no text messaging.[31] Similar studies in children and adolescents with inflammatory bowel disease, recipients of liver transplants, and individuals infected with human immunodeficiency virus revealed increased adherence to medication in individuals who received daily personalized medication reminders via text messaging.[32–34]

Several Web-based text messaging services are available that can provide multiple daily, personalized text messages to remind patients to take their medications (https://www.reminderly.com; https://www.mosio.com). In addition to medication reminders, these programs have the ability to ask for a simple response from the recipient to confirm medication compliance, such as a Y or N (yes or no) text response. In addition, these programs allow patients to text back their own free response, including confirmation of pharmaceutical drug name, dosage, and time taken. Modern text-based software also allows picture messaging if visual medication confirmation is required. In addition, several of these programs have the ability to automatically "nudge" or gently remind the patient to take a medication if the initial text was not confirmed within a specified time frame. Although there are no specific data that exist in the literature related to the use of these apps and the ability to increase medication adherence in patients with portal hypertension and HE specifically, it can be assumed that medication reminders via text messaging would have value in this patient population.

Phone Apps to Remind Patients to Take Their Medications

In addition to text message reminders that prompt patients to take their medications, there are multiple mobile phone apps that serve a similar purpose. A recently published study that analyzed the availability of mobile phone medication adherence apps in 2019 revealed that 704 apps existed, 443 available for Apple devices and 261 for Android, with most being available for both platforms. The investigators noted that the 20 best apps had similar characteristics, including the ability to set up customized medication regimen details and reminders; to monitor other health information, including vital signs and use of supplements; and to support health care visits by sharing this information during visits to providers. However, negative user experiences were reported, including technical difficulties, confusion regarding how to navigate the app, difficulty setting up medication dosage schedules, and inconsistent synchronization of data.[35] Despite these hurdles, there are several studies that indicate improved medication adherence when using mobile phone medication reminder apps, including improved adherence to antiretroviral therapy in men who have sex with men[36] and improved adherence in adolescents with chronic health conditions.[37]

In our practice, we recommend several medication reminder apps to our patients (and ourselves) because they meet several criteria, including:

1. Validation of ease of use by senior citizens
2. Ease of entering medication names, with autocomplete
3. Photographs of the pills/tablets
4. Simplicity related to entering dosing schedules and time of day to take medicine
5. Medicine education for each drug
6. Compliance tracking for family, caregivers, and health care providers
7. Safe rescheduling of missed doses
8. Notification of dangerous drug interactions, which is useful if several different health care providers are prescribing multiple medications
9. Common side effects within the first 24 to 48 hours of starting a new medicine

In addition, several of these apps upload the patient's medication list automatically if the prescription is provided from a CVS, RiteAid, Walgreens, or Walmart pharmacy. Other valuable features include the ability for the patients to upload their copay cards, and information for patient assistance programs for specific medications is suggested. Many of these apps are simple; the name and time to take the medication appears on the patient's phone screen, and patients swipe to confirm that they have taken the medicine, or indicate that they are delaying or skipping a dose. A record is kept on the phone, and family members or caregivers can be automatically notified if the patient misses a medication dose. A valuable additional benefit is that, if patients need to delay taking a medicine because they are not home, a "snooze till home" feature tracks the phone via GPS and reminds the patients to take the medicine when they arrive home. Perhaps most importantly, many of these apps are free.

Automated Medication-Dispensing Technology

Additional medication management technologies include monitored medication-dispensing machines and pill organizers that can safely organize pills/tablets, provide reminders to take medicines, dispense the medications, and notify family members and caregivers of missed doses. These programs are not free, usually requiring a monthly fee; however, there are multiple benefits to these programs. Operationally, the patient gives the pharmacist a medication tray, which is organized using blister packs, and auditory and visual reminders from the pill dispenser allow patients to know which dispenser contains which medications to take at the correct time. In many cases, technologically aware family members can access the medication dispenser schedule remotely via a Web-based interface online. However, most of these systems do not allow liquid medications to be dispensed, which may limit automated dispensing of lactulose. Additional features of these apps can be found at https://www.seniorsafetyreviews.com/reviews/best-medication-reminders/.

Based on the success of mobile phone apps as easily translatable modalities to achieve medication adherence, it is intuitive that these apps could have benefit related to medication adherence in patients with HE. The advantage of these apps is the ability to automate several functions related to medication adherence, including access to medicines; reminders to take medicine; and built-in technology to alert family members, caregivers, and health care providers regarding missed doses, thus potentially minimizing missed doses and HE relapses/exacerbation. The disadvantages of these apps are inherent in the technology; a cellular phone app and text reminder is ineffective if an individual is not able to access the phone or use the app. However, cellular phone use in the United States is pervasive and not limited by education or, in many instances, economic circumstances. Thus, even in technologically challenged individuals, the ability to navigate these apps and text messaging programs should not be an obstacle because the creators of these programs and apps have, in most cases, understood the barriers to use of the technology. **Table 2** lists several technologies that may be valuable to monitor patients with HE.

Telemedicine or Remote Medicine Check-in Visits

In the last several years, it has become apparent that optimal patient care does not always require face-to-face interaction, especially in the setting of chronic disease. Telemedicine offers an opportunity to take advantage of technology to provide on-demand patient care and to perform patient check-ins in a way that is more efficient than traditional office visits. Telemedicine can include a variety of aspects of patient care that can be performed remotely, such as telemonitoring, tele-education, teleconsultation, and telecare, all of which may have value in the setting of HE. Thus, telemedicine seems to be well suited to monitoring and treating patients with HE. Telemonitoring allows health care providers to monitor their patients by using wearable or mobile devices or via Web-based or telephone-based virtual visits to monitor symptoms or disease progression. The signs and symptoms of HE, particularly overt HE, can be easily assessed and evaluated remotely via a Web-based virtual visit. A major component of telemonitoring includes the use of smartphone applications, devices, portals, and social media, and in many cases links to an electronic medical record. Tele-education may be achieved via the use of webinars and interactive sessions that can be accessed by patients and their family members. Patient and family member education regarding the signs and symptoms of HE and treatment can be

Table 2 Technology to enhance medication adherence		
Technique	**Advantage**	**Disadvantage**
Text alert medication reminders	Initiated by clinician Increased medication adherence	Lack of familiarity with technology
Web-based text alert medication reminder	Initiated by clinical team Automated Can confirm that medicine was taken Medication reminders Increased medication adherence	Lack of familiarity with technology Lack of access to phone/Internet
Phone app	Customizable Simple to use Compliance tracking Increased medication adherence	Unwieldy app Technophobe may not be able to use app
Monitored medication-dispensing machines Pill organizers	Organized by pharmacist Automated Notifications if dosing is missed Increased medication adherence	Most cannot dispense liquid

achieved with appropriately focused tele-education sessions. In addition, teleconsultation allows consultation and collaboration between providers and experts who are out of geographic reach; an example of this is the use of teleconsultation in stroke recognition[38] and emergency care situations.[39] The recognition of signs and symptoms and initiation of therapy for HE can be easily established via a remote consultation by a health care provider with experience diagnosing and treating HE.

The aspect of telemedicine that is becoming increasingly appreciated as transformative related to the delivery of medical care is telecare. Telecare is described as video interaction with the patient and health care provider that replicates the face-to-face office visit. There are multiple publications that describe the benefits of telemedicine and telecare in multiple medical specialties, including inflammatory bowel disease,[40] diabetes,[41] and rheumatology.[42] Although there are currently no data to validate the use of telemedicine and telecare in patients with HE, it is clear that the ability to remotely monitor a patient and intervene has significant potential to improve the management of HE via the ability to perform an on-demand or more frequent assessment of patients with HE via virtual visits, and diagnose and treat HE. **Table 3** lists several telemedicine technologies and their applications in HE.

WEARABLE TECHNOLOGY FOR HEPATIC ENCEPHALOPATHY MONITORING

Multiple patient self-monitoring tools exist for a wide range of medical conditions, including blood sugar, blood pressure, and heart rate monitoring, as well as the ability to perform an electrocardiogram. Historically, validated medical devices embedded with sensors have been applied in clinical trials and for targeted research studies conducted in medical settings. However, recent advances in technology now provide the ability to monitor several different activities (eg, steps walked), physiologic parameters (eg, blood oxygen saturation), and biochemical measures (eg, pH). In addition,

Table 3	
Telemedicine in managing hepatic encephalopathy	
Modality	**Potential Uses**
Telemonitoring	Wearable device information can be accessed
Tele-education	Seminars/education sessions with patients and family members related to signs/symptoms of HE and how to treat
Teleconsultation	Providers/patients can provide remote care by working with clinician experts trained in HE management
Telecare	Real-time, on-demand virtual clinician-patient interaction

consumer-accessible wearable technologies are commonly used to track personal wellness, including daily calories burned, number of steps walked, amount of sleep each evening, as well as multiple other parameters. A recent Pew Internet and American Life survey found that 69% of US adults track weight, diet, symptoms, or health routines in some manner (http://www.pewinternet.org/2013/01/28/tracking-for-health).

In addition to the most common wearable devices such as smart watches, there are emerging data regarding the future potential of alternative health trackers, including smart clothing, patches and tattoos, ingestibles, and smart implants (http://rockhealth.com/resources/rock-reports/future-biosensing-wearables).

Wearable technology therefore has the potential for significant benefit related to patient care. Its application has the potential to change and augment the traditional relationship among patients, physicians, and hospitals by facilitating early recognition of a potential untoward health issue, and allow appropriate triaging to determine which patients need to be seen emergently, remotely via telemedicine, or in person via a traditional office visit. There are presently multiple wearable technology applications that are in use, mostly in the cardiology arena, including the ability to measure steps and distance, track vital signs (heart rate, pulse, oximetry, and weight), as well as instantaneous electrocardiogram reading and interpretation with the ability to activate the emergency response system. Wearable technology at present includes smart watches, bracelet-style monitors, and chest-strap devices.[43] In addition, a pilot study using a portable electroencephalography system to monitor patients for changes in their electroencephalograms (EEGs) as a mechanism to assess for HE has recently been published; this technology is being assessed in a larger patient population.[44]

However, there are currently no studies that report the use of wearable technology to allow detection of either CHE or overt HE, although future technology may be developed to achieve this. The potential for these technologies to revolutionize the detection and management of HE is likely significant; next, this article extrapolates what is known about currently available wearable technologies and proposes how future technologies may become useful in the diagnosis and management of HE.

Detection of Signs/Symptoms of Hepatic Encephalopathy

Currently available wearable technology for health monitoring has several valuable attributes in monitoring and diagnosing HE, including an accelerometer and gyroscope for motion detection and an optical sensor for blood flow monitoring. Common applications using this technology are activity tracking via the use of the accelerometer, and heart rate and irregular heart rate monitoring and electrocardiography with the optical sensor. It is therefore feasible that the accelerometer function could be used to assess and monitor for the presence of asterixis, providing a mechanism to alert patients and their health care providers regarding the status of overt HE. It is likely that point-of-care or home recognition of overt HE may allow more rapid initiation of therapy and prompt emergent patient evaluation. An additional component of wearable technology is the ability to detect when a patient falls. The new Apple Watch Series 4 is now classified by the US Food and Drug Administration as a class 2 medical device that not only can perform the functions listed earlier but can also detect when a patient falls. The new accelerometer and gyroscope can measure forces up to $32 \times g$, and analyze wrist trajectory and impact acceleration to determine when a fall occurs. In addition, a phone call to emergency services can be initiated automatically after a fall is detected. This feature, which will presumable be available on additional wearable devices, may be invaluable to assist in detecting advanced HE, because the altered sensorium associated with this condition can lead to falls.

Detection of Serum Ammonia Level

One of the most promising features of smart watches and wearable technology related to future applications in health care is the ability to detect and monitor serum chemistry. At present, several products that provide continuous glucose monitoring are commercially available (https://www.diabetesnet.com/diabetes-technology/meters-monitors/continuous-monitors/compare-current-monitors). A smart watch is being developed that will also provide continuous glucose monitoring, as well as continuous assessment of lactate levels (https://www.pkvitality.com/ktrack). As these and future technology advance, the ability to monitor multiple components of serum, including ammonia levels, can be envisioned. Although serum ammonia level monitoring is a contentious issue in HE, changes in serum ammonia level may predict which patients are at risk of developing progressive HE. It is feasible that future technologies will allow this to become a reality. Wearable smart technology that is currently available and in clinical development and the potential future applications are listed in **Table 4**.

Table 4
Current and future wearable technology and potential application for hepatic encephalopathy

Product	Current Feature	Potential Future Application for HE
Apple Watch	Electrocardiogram, activity tracker, accelerometer measuring asterixis, gyroscope to analyze wrist trajectory and impact to detect falls, automated emergency response	Detection of asterixis Measurement of serum ammonia
K'Watch	In development to monitor serum glucose and lactate	Measurement of serum ammonia
Breitling Emergency	Dual-frequency locator beacon	Patient tracking
Fitbit Ionic	Blood oxygen level saturation measurement being developed	Serum ammonia assessment
Continuous glucose monitors Dexcom Guardian MiniMed Freestyle Libre	Allow continuous blood glucose monitoring	Serum ammonia assessment
Wearable electroencephalography	Detects EEG changes	May provide preemptive diagnosis of HE

SUMMARY

HE is a common manifestation of portal hypertension and cirrhosis, resulting in hospitalizations and readmissions. Prevention of initial hospitalizations as well as readmissions will require a multidisciplinary approach including patient and family education regarding the signs and symptoms of HE, and self-assessment tools that can be used at home by the patients and families to assess for the presence or progression of HE. Enhancing adherence to medication using phone or Web-based text alerts, phone apps, as well as home-based automated medicine-dispensing platforms and pill organizers is paramount. Telemedicine, which can provide remote telemonitoring, patient and family tele-education, on-demand teleconsultation with HE experts, as well as real-time virtual patient-clinician visits, will revolutionize how education, recognition, and treatment of patients with HE occurs. In addition, wearable technology has the future potential to monitor multiple aspects of HE, including asterixis, falls, changes in EEG, and serum ammonia levels, and may allow early recognition and treatment of HE to prevent hospitalization and readmissions.

DISCLOSURE

The authors have nothing to disclose.

REFERENCES

1. Fisher C, Faloon W. Blood ammonia levels in hepatic cirrhosis: their control by the oral administration of neomycin. N Engl J Med 1957;256:1030–5.
2. Conn HO, Leevy CM, Vlahcevic ZR, et al. Comparison of lactulose and neomycin in the treatment of chronic portal-systemic encephalopathy. A double blind controlled trial. Gastroenterology 1977;72:573–83.
3. Bass NM, Mullen KD, Sanyal A, et al. Rifaximin treatment in hepatic encephalopathy. N Engl J Med 2010;362:1071–81.
4. Bajaj JS, Kassam Z, Fagan A, et al. Fecal microbiota transplant from a rational stool donor improves hepatic encephalopathy: a randomized clinical trial. Hepatology 2017;66:1727–38.
5. Tapper EB, Halbert B, Mellinger J. Rates of and reasons for hospital readmissions in patients with cirrhosis: a multistate population-based cohort study. Clin Gastroenterol Hepatol 2016;14:1181–8.
6. Mumtaz K, Issak A, Porter K, et al. Validation of risk score in predicting early readmissions in decompensated cirrhotic patients: a model based on the administrative database. Hepatology 2018. https://doi.org/10.1002/hep.30274.
7. Kruger AJ, Aberra F, Black SM. A validated risk model for prediction of early readmission in patients with hepatic encephalopathy. Ann Hepatol 2019;18:310–7.
8. Vilstrup H, Amodio P, Bajaj J, et al. Hepatic encephalopathy in chronic liver disease: 2014 practice guideline by the European association for the study of the liver and the American Association for the Study of Liver Diseases. Hepatology 2014;60(2):715–35.
9. Neff GW, Kemmer N, Duncan C, et al. Update on the management of cirrhosis - focus on cost-effective preventative strategies. Clinicoecon Outcomes Res 2013; 5:143–52.
10. Stepanova M, Mishra A, Venkatesan C, et al. In-hospital mortality and economic burden associated with hepatic encephalopathy in the United States from 2005 to 2009. Clin Gastroenterol Hepatol 2012;10(9):1034–41.

11. Bustamante J, Rimola A, Ventura PJ, et al. Prognostic significance of hepatic encephalopathy in patients with cirrhosis. J Hepatol 1999;30(5):890–5.

12. Volk ML, Tocco RS, Bazick J, et al. Hospital readmissions among patients with decompensated cirrhosis. Am J Gastroenterol 2012;107:247–52.

13. Saab S. Evaluation of the impact of rehospitalization in the management of hepatic encephalopathy. Int J Gen Med 2015;8:165–73.

14. Chirapongsathorn S, Krittanawong C, Enders F, et al. Incidence and cost analysis of hospital admission and 30-day readmission among patients with cirrhosis. Hepatol Commun 2018;2:188–98.

15. Pantham G, Post A, Venkat D, et al. A new look at precipitants of overt hepatic encephalopathy in cirrhosis. Dig Dis Sci 2017;62:2166–73.

16. Bajaj JS, Sanyal AJ, Bell D, et al. Predictors of the recurrence of hepatic encephalopathy in lactulose-treated patients. Aliment Pharmacol Ther 2010;31:1012–7.

17. Neff G, Zachry W. Systematic review of the economic burden of overt hepatic encephalopathy and pharmacoeconomic impact of rifaximin. Pharmacoeconomics 2018;36(7):809–22.

18. Bajaj JS, Riggio O. Drug therapy: rifaximin. Hepatology 2010;52(4):1484–8.

19. Roggeri DP, Roggeri A. Economic impact of the use of rifaximin 550 mg twice daily for the treatment of overt hepatic encephalopathy in Italy. Hepat Med 2017;9:37–43.

20. Bajaj JS, Pinkerton SD, Sanyal AJ, et al. Diagnosis and treatment of minimal hepatic encephalopathy to prevent motor vehicle accidents: a cost-effectiveness analysis. Hepatology 2012;55(4):1164–71.

21. Leevy CB, Phillips JA. Hospitalizations during the use of rifaximin versus lactulose for the treatment of hepatic encephalopathy. Dig Dis Sci 2007;52(3):737–41.

22. Leise M, Poterucha JJ, Kamat P, et al. Management of hepatic encephalopathy in the hospital. Mayo Clin Proc 2014;89(2):241–53.

23. Neff Guy W, Frederick RT. Assessing treatment patterns in patients with overt hepatic encephalopathy. Hepatology 2012;56(4):945A.

24. Nabi E, Bajaj JS. Useful tests for hepatic encephalopathy in clinical practice. Curr Gastroenterol Rep 2014;16(1):362–8.

25. Bajaj JS, Thacker LR, Heuman DM, et al. The stroop smartphone application is a short and valid method to screen for minimal hepatic encephalopathy. Hepatology 2013;58(3):1122–32.

26. Bajaj JS, Heuman DM, Sterling RK, et al. Validation of EncephalApp, smartphone-based stroop test, for the diagnosis of covert hepatic encephalopathy. Clin Gastroenterol Hepatol 2015;13(10):1828–35.

27. Campagna F, Montagnese S, Ridola L, et al. The animal naming test: an easy tool for the assessment of hepatic encephalopathy. Hepatology 2017;66(1):198–208.

28. Beul L, Toenges G, Ridola L, et al. Validation of the simplified Animal Naming Test as primary screening tool for the diagnosis of covert hepatic encephalopathy. Eur J Intern Med 2019;60:96–100.

29. Tapper EB, Parikh ND, Waljee AK, et al. Diagnosis of minimal hepatic encephalopathy: a systematic review of point-of-care diagnostic tests. Am J Gastroenterol 2018;113(4):529–38.

30. Chisholm-Burns MA, Spivey CA. The "cost" of medication nonadherence: consequences we cannot afford to accept. J Am Pharm Assoc 2012;52(6):823–6.

31. Thakkar J, Kurup R, Laba TL, et al. Mobile telephone text messaging for medication adherence in chronic disease: a meta-analysis. JAMA Intern Med 2016; 176(3):340–9.

32. Miloh T, Shub M, Montes R, et al. Text messaging effect on adherence in children with inflammatory bowel disease. J Pediatr Gastroenterol Nutr 2017;64(6): 939–42.

33. Miloh T, Annunziato R, Arnon R, et al. Improved adherence and outcomes for pediatric liver transplant recipients by using text messaging. Pediatrics 2009; 124(5):e844–50.

34. Horvath T, Azman H, Kennedy GE, et al. Mobile phone text messaging for promoting adherence to antiretroviral therapy in patients with HIV infection. Cochrane Database Syst Rev 2012;(3):1–49.

35. Park JYE, Li J, Howren A, et al. Mobile phone apps targeting medication adherence: quality assessment and content analysis of user reviews. JMIR Mhealth Uhealth 2019;7(1):1–11.

36. Muessig KE, LeGrand S, Horvath KJ, et al. Recent mobile health interventions to support medication adherence among HIV-positive MSM. Curr Opin HIV AIDS 2017;12(5):432–41.

37. Badawy SM, Barrera L, Sinno MG, et al. Text messaging and mobile phone apps as interventions to improve adherence in adolescents with chronic health conditions: a systematic review. JMIR Mhealth Uhealth 2017;5(5):66–71.

38. Schwamm LH, Holloway RG, Amarenco P, et al. A review of the evidence for the use of telemedicine within stroke systems of care: a scientific statement from the American Heart Association/American Stroke Association. Stroke 2009;40: 2616–34.

39. Ward MM, Jaana M, Natafgi N. Systematic review of telemedicine applications in emergency rooms. Int J Med Inform 2015;84:601–16.

40. Aguas Peris M, Del Hoyo J, Bebia P, et al. Telemedicine in inflammatory bowel disease: opportunities and approaches. Inflamm Bowel Dis 2015;21:392–9.

41. Huang Z, Tao H, Meng Q, et al. Management of endocrine disease. Effects of telecare intervention on glycemic control in type 2 diabetes: a systematic review and meta-analysis of randomized controlled trials European. J Endocrinol 2015; 172:93–101.

42. El Miedanye Y. e-Rheumatology: are we ready? Clin Rheumatol 2015;34:831–7.

43. Foster KR, Torous J. The opportunity and obstacles for smartwatches and wearable sensors. IEEE Pulse 2019;10:22–5.

44. Zhang Q, Wang P, Liu Y, et al. A real-time wireless wearable electroencephalography system based on Support Vector Machine for encephalopathy daily monitoring. Int J Distrib Sens Netw 2018;14:1–9.

Social Impact of Hepatic Encephalopathy

Mishal Reja, MD[a],*, Lauren Pioppo Phelan, MD[a], Frank Senatore, MD[b],
Vinod K. Rustgi, MD, MBA[c],*

KEYWORDS

- Quality of life • Driving • Sleep • Finance • Caregiver • Social impact

KEY POINTS

- For patients with HE, activities of daily living including sleep, mobility, work, and driving have been demonstrated to be significantly affected.
- Multiple tools are available to assess quality of life challenges, including the CLD-Q questionnaire.
- Hepatic encephalopathy also presents a significant financial burden to patients and families through work capacity and caregiver burden.
- Both rifaximin and lactulose have been shown to improve quality of life and social impacts.

INTRODUCTION

Hepatic encephalopathy (HE) is a multifaceted disorder, with its effects stretching far beyond office visits and hospitalizations. There are many social factors affected in a patient's life with HE. These factors are extremely underrecognized and have the potential to harbor dangerous, life-altering consequences. Social impacts of HE revolve around a patient's quality of life (QoL) and include their work capacity, driving ability, and sleep quality. The burden on their caregiver is equally affected, posing additional challenges.

QUALITY OF LIFE

Patients with HE suffer from varying degrees of altered consciousness, intellectual disability, and personality changes that severely impact their QoL.[1] The World Health Organization defines QoL as "the individuals' perception of their position in life in the context of the culture and value system in which they live and in relation to their goals, standards, and concerns."[2] Health-related QoL (HRQoL) indicates the subjective

[a] Department of Medicine, Rutgers Robert Wood Johnson University Hospital, Clinical Academic Building (CAB), 125 Paterson Street, Suite 5100B, New Brunswick, NJ 08901, USA; [b] Department of Gastroenterology, Rutgers Robert Wood Johnson University Hospital, Clinical Academic Building, 125 Paterson Street, Suite 5100B, New Brunswick, NJ 08901, USA; [c] Center for Liver Diseases and Masses, Robert Wood Johnson Medical School, Clinical Academic Building (CAB), 125 Paterson Street, Suite 5100B, New Brunswick, NJ 08901, USA
* Corresponding authors.
E-mail addresses: dr845@rwjms.rutgers.edu (M.R.); vr262@rwjms.rutgers.edu (V.K.R.)

Clin Liver Dis 24 (2020) 291–301
https://doi.org/10.1016/j.cld.2020.01.008
1089-3261/20/© 2020 Elsevier Inc. All rights reserved.

perception of QoL in relation to acute and chronic disease based on physical, psychological, and social functioning.[3] Given that QoL has been shown to be more important to patients than their longevity, evaluating HRQoL has gained an integral role in medical treatment.[4]

There is no single best measurement to assess HRQoL in HE, although there are multiple modalities available. HRQoL is most commonly measured by using general health scales, such as the Sickness Impact Profile (SIP), the Nottingham Health Profile (NHP), Medical Outcomes Study Short Form-36 (SF-36), and the Chronic Liver Disease Questionnaire (CLD-Q) (**Table 1**). The SIP consists of 136 items grouped into 12 categories. It is used to assess the influence of HE on daily functioning and takes several minutes to perform; however, its main limitation is that patients with cognitive dysfunction may fail to complete the entire questionnaire.[5] The NHP is a two-part questionnaire that measures distress, but is less sensitive to subtle changes in HE.[6,7] The SF-36 includes 36 items that cover health status across eight domains.[8,9] It is most frequently used in clinical practice because of its ease of use and good sensitivity. CLD-Q is a questionnaire assessing QoL in chronic liver disease.[10] It is the most widely used of all the questionnaires because of its conciseness, allowing for timely assessments. Its main limitation is that its sensitivity decreases with worsening of liver disease.

Most studies analyzing HRQoL in HE have focused on minimal HE (MHE), the mildest form of HE. This is because overt HE (OHE) is often difficult to assess during an acute episode because of a patient's impaired consciousness. MHE is characterized by subtle cognitive and psychomotor deficits in the absence of recognizable clinical symptoms.[11] The neurocognitive abnormalities affected are primarily attention, information processing, visuospatial abilities, and psychomotor coordination. Complex activities, such as driving a car or learning a complex topic, can be impaired, whereas basic functions, such as personal hygiene or verbal abilities, are normally preserved.[12]

There are several small studies that exist evaluating HRQoL in patients with OHE and MHE. A study of 160 patients with cirrhosis found that HE had a profound effect on HRQoL, and the degree of HE determined the extent to which HRQoL was impacted. OHE had a significant effect on physical and mental domains of SF-36, whereas MHE had significant effects on mental and emotional domains.[9]

Table 1
Health scales for HRQoL

SIP	NHP	SF-36	CLD-Q
Sleep and rest	Part 1: Present distress	Physical functioning	Abdominal symptoms
Eating	Energy	Physical role limitation	Fatigue
Work	Sleep	Bodily pain	Systemic symptoms
Home management	Pain	General health	Activity
Recreation and	Emotional reactions	Emotional role	Emotional function
pastimes	Social isolation	limitation	Worry
Ambulation	Physical mobility	Vitality	
Mobility	Part 2: Everyday	Mental health	
Body care and	activities	Social functioning	
movement	Occupation		
Social interactions	Jobs		
Alertness behavior	Home		
Emotional behavior	Social life		
Communication	Home life		
	Sex life		
	Hobbies		
	Holidays		

MHE has been directly correlated to adverse effects on HRQoL.[13-16] Hartmann and colleagues[14] examined 79 patients and found that low SIP scores were significantly linked to MHE in the domains of alertness, sleep and rest, fine motor skills, and work.[17] Bao and colleagues[18] examined 106 patients with MHE and found that SF-36 scores were lower in MHE, although no differences were shown in CLD-Q scores. In 554 patients with cirrhosis, the presence of OHE and MHE affected physical and mental aspects of SF-36 and NHP across all domains except pain.[13]

On the contrary, a few studies did not demonstrate significant effects of MHE on HRQoL. Tan and colleagues[19] studied 36 patients in a short-term prospective trial and found that HRQoL was still impaired after resolution of MHE, suggesting that MHE was not the responsible underlying factor. Nevertheless, the authors postulated that given most patients in this study had viral cirrhosis, this may independently reduce HRQoL resulting in their findings. Another study by Wunsch and colleagues[17] found that SF-36 and CLD-Q scores were not significantly different between patients with or without MHE. Despite this, this study was poorly powered and its small sample size likely resulted in selection bias.

Several treatments for MHE have been shown to improve HRQoL, which associates causality to MHE. Prasad and colleagues[20] enrolled 90 patients with cirrhosis with MHE and treated them with 3 months of lactulose therapy. They showed a significant improvement in HRQoL on several SIP domains, including emotion behavior, sleep, recreation, mobility, and pastimes. However, a subsequent meta-analysis failed to show that lactulose improved HRQoL.[21] In a study of 284 patients with cirrhosis treated with 8 weeks of rifaximin, MHE significantly improved psychometric and SIP scores, and driving and cognitive performance.[22] These results were confirmed in a randomized controlled trial that showed significantly improved HRQoL in patients taking rifaximin.[22] Thus far, randomized controlled trials evaluating probiotics have not been shown to improve MHE or HRQoL.[23]

WORK CAPACITY

Employment status and earning ability is important for livelihood and personal satisfaction, and impairment in working ability can negatively affect HRQoL. Global intelligence and verbal ability is preserved in MHE, whereas psychomotor functions are impaired.[22] As a result, patients with MHE in occupations that require psychomotor coordination had reduced HRQoL. To investigate this, Schomerus and colleagues[24] evaluated 110 patients with cirrhosis in Germany in the ambulatory care setting. He demonstrated that blue-collar workers (drivers, carpenters, factory workers) were primary affected by HE as opposed to white-collar workers (doctors, lawyers, academicians). Sixty percent of blue-collar workers were considered unfit to work by the German social security system versus only 20% of white-collar workers.[24] Additionally, half of the patients with MHE were unemployed versus only 15% without MHE. Psychometric tests were similar in unemployed and employed cohorts with the exception of psychomotor function, which was more prevalent in unemployed patients. Blue-collar workers had a higher prevalence of alcoholism, which may have independently decreased HRQoL.

More recently, Bajaj and colleagues[25] evaluated 104 patients with cirrhosis of whom 44% had previous episodes of HE. Forty-four percent stopped working after the diagnosis of cirrhosis, although 71% reported they would work if they were able too. Fifty-three percent of patients decreased their work hours, 56% of families stopped saving because of medical costs, 46% incurred debt, 11% did not have enough money for food, and 7% went into bankruptcy.[25] This study highlighted the progressive financial deterioration that HE can cause in a patient's life.

IMPLICATIONS FOR DRIVING

The neurocognitive dysfunction typical of OHE and MHE may also have a significant impact on a patient's ability to drive safely. Multiple skills are necessary for safe driving including attention, working memory, and psychomotor coordination.[26] These abilities can all be severely impaired in HE. Although it seems apparent that patients with OHE are too neurocognitively impaired to drive, it is less clear for those with MHE. Studies across several countries have demonstrated that patients with MHE have delayed reaction time when driving, and one study showed that these patients required more prompting and interventions by a driving instructor to prevent accidents.[26–29] During on-road driving tests, patients with cirrhosis with MHE have been found to have significantly poorer car handling, adaptation, and cautiousness compared with patients with cirrhosis without MHE.[29] It has also been specifically demonstrated that those with MHE have impaired navigation skills and are more likely to make illegal turns.[30]

It is well documented that patients with MHE seem to have deficits in skills essential to safe driving (**Fig. 1**). Because traffic accidents represent one of the leading causes of death worldwide, it is critical to determine whether MHE poses a danger to themselves or others on the road. There is evidence to suggest that these patients do have worse driving outcomes, including increased traffic accidents and violations, compared with those without HE. However, these results were based on anonymous driving outcomes questionnaires, and therefore prospective studies are needed to verify these data.[31] A more recent study showed that patients with MHE had significantly more collisions and performed worse on driving simulators with increasing fatigue compared with those without HE.[32]

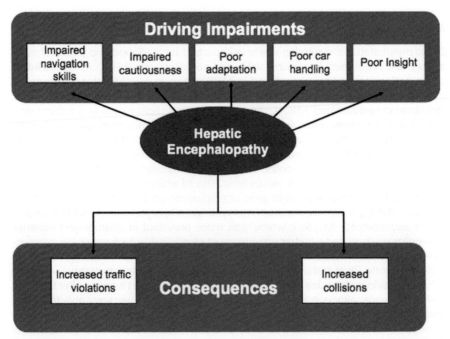

Fig. 1. Driving deficits of those with hepatic encephalopathy and their potential real-life consequences.

Although evidence supporting poor driving outcomes in those with MHE is limited, the potential danger that this disease poses on driving suggests that including driving history in regular evaluations of patients with cirrhosis may be beneficial. In addition to the documented impaired driving skills, one study demonstrated that patients with MHE seem to lack insight into their driving skills.[33] Thus, not only are these people poor drivers, but they also seem to be unaware of their own deficits. This suggests that providers should consider taking a full driving history from the patient and from another reliable source that is exposed to the patient's driving skills.[34]

When those with MHE do suffer from a motor vehicle accident, they seem to have worse outcomes than those without cirrhosis, especially those with a high Child-Pugh score. These patients generally do worse than normal control subjects after any trauma or surgery.[35] These poor outcomes after motor vehicle accidents include longer hospital stays and, most importantly, higher mortality rates.[36] Thus, those with cirrhosis and HE may be more likely to get into a traffic accident and subsequently have higher mortality rates after an accident. This again highlights the importance of taking an accurate driving history and advising driving restrictions in those with MHE.

It is unclear whether treatment of MHE improves driving outcomes. One small randomized placebo control study did find that patients treated with rifaximin have improved performance on driving simulators than those taking placebo.[22] However, further evidence for treatment of HE leading to better driving is limited.

Overall, it seems that those with MHE have neurocognitive deficits that are fundamental to safe driving. There is evidence that these deficits may lead to increased traffic violations and motor vehicle accidents, and importantly, that these patients lack insight into these deficits and are unaware of their poor driving. Thus, providers should consider taking a comprehensive and accurate driving history to assess the patient's safety on the road and potentially limit their driving if necessary.

SLEEP DISTURBANCE

Sleep disturbances are well documented in those with cirrhosis, and they tend to be more common in those with MHE compared with those without.[20,37–41] Generally, sleep disturbance tends to be an early sign of HE, and this disturbance can further worsen neuropsychiatric impairment.[41,42] However, the evidence for this is inconsistent, and other studies have suggested that sleep disturbance is unrelated to the presence or absence of HE.[39] Thus, the relationship between HE and sleep disturbance needs to be further elucidated.

Disturbance of sleep in those with cirrhosis is caused by multiple factors including fatigue, pruritus, poor sleep hygiene, medications, and pain and discomfort associated with the disease itself. However, it may also be a direct consequence of liver dysfunction (**Fig. 2**).[43] Although the mechanism underlying this sleep disturbance is largely unknown, it may be related to circadian rhythm dysfunction. Disruption of melatonin metabolism likely plays a significant role, because melatonin is metabolized by the liver. Patients with cirrhosis have been found to have higher levers of daytime melatonin than nighttime, and there is also a delay in the onset of the peak nocturnal plasma melatonin level.[44] Overall, this suggests that patients with cirrhosis may have delayed sleep onset, and this delayed peak of melatonin secretion is associated with the degree of liver failure.[45–48]

Multiple studies have confirmed delayed sleep onset and poor sleep quality in patients with cirrhosis.[37,39,47] However, another hallmark feature of sleep disturbance in these patients is excessive daytime sleepiness.[37,39–41] This increased daytime fatigue can impair daytime functioning and has been shown to decrease overall QoL.[44,49,50] Excessive daytime fatigue may play a role in a patient's ability to maintain

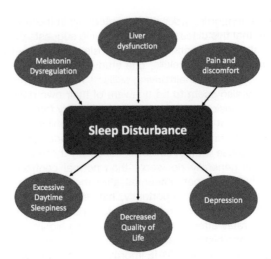

Fig. 2. Various factors causing sleep disturbance in hepatic encephalopathy and its consequences.

a job, drive safely, and complete activities of daily living. Importantly, these sleep disturbances also seem to contribute to increased psychological distress and depression, which can further decrease QoL.[38]

Other sleep disorders, such as obstructive sleep apnea and restless legs syndrome, are also associated with cirrhosis and may contribute to overall sleep disturbance in these patients.[51,52] In those with obstructive sleep apnea and liver cirrhosis, continuous positive airway pressure has been shown to significantly improve executive function and sleep quality.[53] Additionally, in those with alcohol misuse disorder and cirrhosis, alcohol consumption also negatively effects the sleep-wake cycle, with prolonged alcohol misuse causing severe insomnia, altered sleep architecture, and excessive daytime sleepiness.[54,55] Furthermore, in those attempting to achieve sobriety, abstinence from alcohol can unfortunately lead to protracted sleep disruption with insomnia and sleep fragmentation, and is predictive of relapse.[56]

If sleep disturbance is correlated with HE, then it is reasonable to suggest that treatment of HE may improve sleep quality. There is evidence that adequate treatment with lactulose does improve sleep quality and QoL, but rifaximin does not seem to improve sleep quality or daytime sleepiness.[57,58] There are no current studies that have investigated the effect of probiotics on sleep disturbance in this patient population. Thus, further studies are needed to determine if the treatment of HE may improve quality of sleep.

BURDEN ON THE CAREGIVER

Although it is well demonstrated that cirrhosis decreases QoL of the patient, the burden on the family and caregivers of the patient has not been well established. Given the extent of care that a patient with cirrhosis may require, it is reasonable to suggest that the caregiver may suffer from emotional and socioeconomic burdens. Caregivers are often required to make sacrifices to care for the patient, absorb medical costs, and ensure that the patient is compliant with medical therapy. This is an especially important subject, because a good social support system is required for patients to be a candidate for liver transplantation.[25] One study of a small cohort of patients with cirrhosis found that the disease imposes significant financial, socioeconomic, and personal burden on caregivers, and this burden increases with severity of liver disease. The emotional and social burden of the caregiver also increased when the patient had HE, and financial strains were often worsened because of the patient's inability to work.[25] Personal income and employment decrease with worsening cognitive performance of these patients, and this is independent of education level.[59]

Many studies have revealed the financial burden on caregivers of those with chronic disease, and these burdens may increase depression and even mortality in the caregiver.[60–64] A study that interviewed caregivers of patients on the liver transplant list revealed that many family members reported feeling uninformed and unprepared for the consequences of liver disease. Families reported an overall poor understanding of the disease, and demonstrated a lack of knowledge of the relationship between symptoms and the disease process.[63] Another study reported that 19% of caregivers of patients awaiting a kidney or liver transplant reported symptoms of depression.[63]

Thus, although the burden on families and caregivers of those with cirrhosis has not been clearly defined, there is evidence to suggest that these families suffer from social and economic burdens, and these stressors can lead to increased rates of depression and even mortality in the caregiver population. Given the integral role that caregivers play in the management of these patients and the requirement of a strong social support system for liver transplant listing, it is important for providers to address the needs of the caregiver and family.

SUMMARY

The social impacts of HE are becoming more and more apparent in society. OHE and MHE have been shown to adversely affect overall QoL and HRQoL. Specifically, activities of daily living including sleep, mobility, work, and driving have been demonstrated to be significantly impacted in these patient populations. Accurately assessing factors, such as QoL, presents challenges, but there are multiple tools available including the CLD-Q, which offers care providers a simple modality with potential profound benefits.

Specific social factors with well-documented impacts from HE include driving ability and sleep quality. HE has been shown to clearly affect a patient's ability to drive, and their ability to perceive these limitations. This lack of insight is detrimental; therefore, taking a detailed driving history and implementing driving restrictions when applicable is vital. Evidence is also growing that sleep disturbances are mechanistically linked to patients with cirrhosis via a circadian rhythm disorder and associations with restless leg syndrome. These sleep disturbances include delayed sleep onset, poor sleep quality, and excessive daytime sleepiness and sleep apnea.

HE can also present a significant financial burden to patients and families. Work capacity, a noteworthy contributor to overall financial stability in any person, is substantially limited in patients with HE. Caregiver burden is another real issue in patients with HE. Both depression and financial burden have been directly linked to caregivers of patients with cirrhosis with HE. It is essential that all evaluations of patients with HE include simultaneously addressing caregivers.

Common treatments for HE have been shown to improve QoL by directly improving HE. Rifaximin has growing evidence of potential benefits to improve overall QoL and driving performance. Similarly, lactulose may improve overall sleep quality and overall QoL. These findings are promising, although prospective research is required to further substantiate these findings. The most important thing that care providers can immediately implement are detailed evaluations that include screening and evaluation tools to identify the social impacts of HE.

DISCLOSURES

The authors have nothing to disclose.

REFERENCES

1. Arguedas MR, DeLawrence TG, McGuire BM. Influence of hepatic encephalopathy on health-related quality of life in patients with cirrhosis. Dig Dis Sci 2003; 48(8):1622–6.
2. Development of the World Health Organization WHOQOL-BREF quality of life assessment. The WHOQOL Group. Psychol Med 1998;28(3):551–8.
3. Aaronson NK. Quality of life: what is it? How should it be measured? Oncology (Williston Park) 1988;2(5):69–76, 64.
4. McNeil BJ, Weichselbaum R, Pauker SG. Speech and survival: tradeoffs between quality and quantity of life in laryngeal cancer. N Engl J Med 1981;305(17):982–7.
5. Bergner M, Bobbitt RA, Carter WB, et al. The Sickness Impact Profile: development and final revision of a health status measure. Med Care 1981;19(8): 787–805.
6. Hunt SM, McKenna SP, McEwen J, et al. A quantitative approach to perceived health status: a validation study. J Epidemiol Community Health 1980;34(4): 281–6.
7. Hunt SM, McEwen J, McKenna SP. Measuring health status: a new tool for clinicians and epidemiologists. J R Coll Gen Pract 1985;35(273):185–8.
8. Ware JE, Sherbourne CD. The MOS 36-item short-form health survey (SF-36). I. Conceptual framework and item selection. Med Care 1992;30(6):473–83.
9. Brazier JE, Harper R, Jones NM, et al. Validating the SF-36 health survey questionnaire: new outcome measure for primary care. BMJ 1992;305(6846):160–4.
10. Younossi ZM, Guyatt G, Kiwi M, et al. Development of a disease specific questionnaire to measure health related quality of life in patients with chronic liver disease. Gut 1999;45(2):295–300.
11. Dhiman RK, Saraswat VA, Sharma BK, et al. Minimal hepatic encephalopathy: consensus statement of a working party of the Indian National Association for Study of the Liver. J Gastroenterol Hepatol 2010;25(6):1029–41.
12. Ortiz M, Córdoba J, Jacas C, et al. Neuropsychological abnormalities in cirrhosis include learning impairment. J Hepatol 2006;44(1):104–10.
13. Marchesini G, Bianchi G, Amodio P, et al. Factors associated with poor health-related quality of life of patients with cirrhosis. Gastroenterology 2001;120(1): 170–8.
14. Hartmann IJ, Groeneweg M, Quero JC, et al. The prognostic significance of subclinical hepatic encephalopathy. Am J Gastroenterol 2000;95(8):2029–34.
15. Schomerus H, Hamster W. Quality of life in cirrhotics with minimal hepatic encephalopathy. Metab Brain Dis 2001;16(1–2):37–41.
16. Gentilini P, Laffi G, La Villa G, et al. Long course and prognostic factors of virus-induced cirrhosis of the liver. Am J Gastroenterol 1997;92(1):66–72.
17. Wunsch E, Szymanik B, Post M, et al. Minimal hepatic encephalopathy does not impair health-related quality of life in patients with cirrhosis: a prospective study. Liver Int 2011;31(7):980–4.

18. Bao ZJ, Qiu DK, Ma X, et al. The application of psychometric measures in diagnosis of minimal hepatic encephalopathy. Zhonghua Xiaohua Zazhi 2006;26:606–9.

19. Tan HH, Lee GH, Thia KTJ, et al. Minimal hepatic encephalopathy runs a fluctuating course: results from a three-year prospective cohort follow-up study. Singapore Med J 2009;50(3):255–60.

20. Prasad S, Dhiman RK, Duseja A, et al. Lactulose improves cognitive functions and health-related quality of life in patients with cirrhosis who have minimal hepatic encephalopathy. Hepatology 2007;45(3):549–59.

21. Gluud LL, Vilstrup H, Morgan MY. Non-absorbable disaccharides versus placebo/no intervention and lactulose versus lactitol for the prevention and treatment of hepatic encephalopathy in people with cirrhosis. Cochrane Database Syst Rev 2016;(4):CD003044.

22. Bajaj JS, Heuman DM, Wade JB, et al. Rifaximin improves driving simulator performance in a randomized trial of patients with minimal hepatic encephalopathy. Gastroenterology 2011;140(2):478–87.

23. Bajaj JS, Saeian K, Christensen KM, et al. Probiotic yogurt for the treatment of minimal hepatic encephalopathy. Am J Gastroenterol 2008;103(7):1707–15.

24. Schomerus H, Hamster W. Quality of life in cirrhotics with minimal hepatic encephalopathy. Metab Brain Dis 2001;16(1–2):37–41.

25. Bajaj JS, Wade JB, Gibson DP, et al. The multi-dimensional burden of cirrhosis and hepatic encephalopathy on patients and caregivers. Am J Gastroenterol 2011;106(9):1646–53.

26. Evans L. The dominant role of driver behavior in traffic safety. Am J Public Health 1996;86(6):784–6.

27. Poordad FF. Review article: the burden of hepatic encephalopathy. Aliment Pharmacol Ther 2007;1:3–9.

28. Watanabe A, Tuchida T, Yata Y, et al. Evaluation of neuropsychological function in patients with liver cirrhosis with special reference to their driving ability. Metab Brain Dis 1995;10(3):239–48.

29. Wein C, Koch H, Popp B, et al. Minimal hepatic encephalopathy impairs fitness to drive. Hepatology 2004;39(3):739–45.

30. Bajaj JS, Hafeezullah M, Hoffmann RG, et al. Navigation skill impairment: another dimension of the driving difficulties in minimal hepatic encephalopathy. Hepatology 2008;47:596–604.

31. Bajaj JS, Hafeezullah M, Hoffmann RG, et al. Minimal hepatic encephalopathy: a vehicle for accidents and traffic violations. Am J Gastroenterol 2007;102:1903–9.

32. Bajaj JS, Hafeezullah M, Zadvornova Y, et al. The effect of fatigue on driving skills in patients with hepatic encephalopathy. Am J Gastroenterol 2009;104:898–905.

33. Bajaj JS, Saeian K, Hafeezullah M, et al. Patients with minimal hepatic encephalopathy have poor insight into their driving skills. Clin Gastroenterol Hepatol 2008;6:1135–9 [quiz: 1065].

34. Bajaj JS. Minimal hepatic encephalopathy matters in daily life. World J Gastroenterol 2008;14:3609–15.

35. Teh SH, Nagorney DM, Stevens SR, et al. Risk factors for mortality after surgery in patients with cirrhosis. Gastroenterology 2007;132:1261–9.

36. Bajaj JS, Ananthakrishnan AN, McGinley EL, et al. Deleterious effect of cirrhosis on outcomes after motor vehicle crashes using the nationwide inpatient sample. Am J Gastroenterol 2008;103:1674–81.

37. Córdoba J, Cabrera J, Lataif L, et al. High prevalence of sleep disturbance in cirrhosis. Hepatology 1998;27:339–45.

38. Bianchi G, Marchesini G, Nicolino F, et al. Psychological status and depression in patients with liver cirrhosis. Dig Liver Dis 2005;37:593–600.
39. Montagnese S, Middleton B, Skene DJ, et al. Night-time sleep disturbance does not correlate with neuropsychiatric impairment in patients with cirrhosis. Liver Int 2009;29:1372–82.
40. Mostacci B, Ferlisi M, Baldi Antognini A, et al. Sleep disturbance and daytime sleepiness in patients with cirrhosis: a case control study. Neurol Sci 2008;29: 237–40.
41. Samanta J, Dhiman RK, Khatri A, et al. Correlation between degree and quality of sleep disturbance and the level of neuropsychiatric impairment in patients with liver cirrhosis. Metab Brain Dis 2013;28:249–59.
42. Sherlock S, Summerskill WH, White LP, et al. Portal-systemic encephalopathy; neurological complications of liver disease. Lancet 1954;267:454–7.
43. Formentin C, Garrido M, Montagnese S. Assessment and management of sleep disturbance in cirrhosis. Curr Hepatol Rep 2018;17:52–69.
44. Montagnese S, De Pittà C, De Rui M, et al. Sleep-wake abnormalities in patients with cirrhosis. Hepatology 2014;59:705–12.
45. Moore-Ede MC, Czeisler CA, Richardson GS. Circadian timekeeping in health and disease. Part 2. Clinical implications of circadian rhythmicity. N Engl J Med 1983;309:530–6.
46. Disruption of the diurnal rhythm of plasma melatonin in cirrhosis. Available at: https://www.ncbi.nlm.nih.gov/pubmed/7611593. Accessed January 11, 2019.
47. Montagnese S, Middleton B, Mani AR, et al. Sleep and circadian abnormalities in patients with cirrhosis: features of delayed sleep phase syndrome? Metab Brain Dis 2009;24:427–39.
48. Montagnese S, Middleton B, Mani AR, et al. On the origin and the consequences of circadian abnormalities in patients with cirrhosis. Am J Gastroenterol 2010;105: 1773–81.
49. Heeren M, Sojref F, Schuppner R, et al. Active at night, sleepy all day: sleep disturbances in patients with hepatitis C virus infection. J Hepatol 2014;60:732–40.
50. Ghabril M, Jackson M, Gotur R, et al. Most individuals with advanced cirrhosis have sleep disturbances, which are associated with poor quality of life. Clin Gastroenterol Hepatol 2017;15:1271–8.e6.
51. Chou T-C, Liang W-M, Wang C-B, et al. Obstructive sleep apnea is associated with liver disease: a population-based cohort study. Sleep Med 2015;16:955–60.
52. Franco RA, Ashwathnarayan R, Deshpandee A, et al. The high prevalence of restless legs syndrome symptoms in liver disease in an academic-based hepatology practice. J Clin Sleep Med 2008;4:45–9.
53. Effects of obstructive sleep apnea on sleep quality, cognition, and driving performance in patients with cirrhosis. Available at: https://www.ncbi.nlm.nih.gov/pubmed/25158922/. Accessed January 13, 2019.
54. Brower KJ, Perron BE. Sleep disturbance as a universal risk factor for relapse in addictions to psychoactive substances. Med Hypotheses 2010;74:928–33.
55. Colrain IM, Turlington S, Baker FC. Impact of alcoholism on sleep architecture and EEG power spectra in men and women. Sleep 2009;32:1341–52.
56. Thakkar MM, Sharma R, Sahota P. Alcohol disrupts sleep homeostasis. Alcohol 2015;49:299–310.
57. Singh J, Sharma BC, Puri V, et al. Sleep disturbances in patients of liver cirrhosis with minimal hepatic encephalopathy before and after lactulose therapy. Metab Brain Dis 2017;32:595–605.

58. Bruyneel M, Sersté T, Libert W, et al. Improvement of sleep architecture parameters in cirrhotic patients with recurrent hepatic encephalopathy with the use of rifaximin. Eur J Gastroenterol Hepatol 2017;29:302–8.
59. Bajaj JS, Riggio O, Allampati S, et al. Cognitive dysfunction is associated with poor socioeconomic status in patients with cirrhosis: an international multicenter study. Clin Gastroenterol Hepatol 2013;11:1511–6.
60. Schulz R, Beach SR. Caregiving as a risk factor for mortality: the caregiver health effects study. JAMA 1999;282:2215–9.
61. Sherwood PR, Given CW, Given BA, et al. Caregiver burden and depressive symptoms: analysis of common outcomes in caregivers of elderly patients. J Aging Health 2005;17:125–47.
62. Cohen M, Katz D, Baruch Y. Stress among the family caregivers of liver transplant recipients. Prog Transplant 2007;17:48–53.
63. Bolkhir A, Loiselle MM, Evon DM, et al. Depression in primary caregivers of patients listed for liver or kidney transplantation. Prog Transplant 2007;17: 193–8.
64. Miyazaki ET, Dos Santos R, Miyazaki MC, et al. Patients on the waiting list for liver transplantation: caregiver burden and stress. Liver Transpl 2010; 16:1164–8.

Novel Therapies in Hepatic Encephalopathy

Maryam Alimirah, MD[a], Omar Sadiq, MD[b], Stuart C. Gordon, MD[b,c],*

KEYWORDS

- Hepatic encephalopathy • Ammonia scavengers • Glycerolphenylbutyrate
- Polyethylene glycol • Acetyl-L-carnitine • Flumazenil • Gut

KEY POINTS

- The gold standard for treatment of hepatic encephalopathy with lactulose and rifaxmin has shortcomings with regards to efficacy and compliance.
- Ammonia-scavenging agents, such as L-ornithine phenylacetate and glycerol glycerolphenylbutyrate demonstrate decrease in ammonia levels and improved cognition in hepatic encephalopathy.
- The gut microbiome is a promising target for ameliorating the effect of hepatic encephalopathy as shown by studies using fecal microbiota transplantation and probiotics.

INTRODUCTION

The aim of current therapies for hepatic encephalopathy (HE) is to increase quality of life by improving mentation and decreasing the rates of hospital admissions related to this complication of decompensated cirrhosis. The current standard of care and the only therapies US Food and Drug Administration approved for treatment of HE include oral lactulose and rifaximin.

Lactulose, a disaccharide probiotic, acidifies the stool, resulting in conversion of gut ammonia (NH_3) to nonabsorbable ammonia cation (NH_4+) and facilitating its subsequent excretion through the gut by catharsis. Rifaximin is an antibiotic that may be added for those who do not respond to lactulose monotherapy; it alters the gut flora and decreases the burden of urease-producing bacteria, which are involved in the pathophysiology of HE. Both of these agents are also thought to reverse possible precipitants of encephalopathy, such as infection, electrolyte abnormalities, gastrointestinal bleeding, and dehydration.

Funding sources: None.
[a] Department of Internal Medicine, Henry Ford Hospital, 2799 West Grand Boulevard, CFP-1, Detroit, MI 48202, USA; [b] Department of Gastroenterology and Hepatology, Henry Ford Hospital, 2799 West Grand Boulevard, K7, Detroit, MI 48202, USA; [c] Wayne State University School of Medicine, Detroit, MI, USA
* Corresponding author. Department of Gastroenterology and Hepatology, Henry Ford Hospital, 2799 West Grand Boulevard, K7, Detroit, MI 48202.
E-mail address: sgordon3@hfhs.org

Despite the widespread use of lactulose and rifaximin, HE remains a major burden in the cirrhotic population due to the high rate of recurrence. An estimated 40% of patients with cirrhosis suffer recurrent episodes of HE despite treatment with lactulose[1] and 1-month readmission rates for HE are as high as 37%.[2,3] Furthermore, adherence to lactulose therapy is hindered by its unpalatable taste and associated gastrointestinal complaints.[4]

In previous decades, alternative HE treatment agents included use of antimicrobials, such as neomycin and metronidazole, but these were largely abandoned due to unfavorable toxicity profiles, including ototoxicity and neurotoxicity, respectively. These limitations have provided the impetus to develop novel treatment modalities for HE—particularly given that options for treating HE not responsive to lactulose and rifaximin are limited in the United States. Fortunately, there are many novel therapies emerging (**Table 1**).

AMMONIA SCAVENGERS
L-Ornithine Phenylacetate and L-Ornithine-L-Aspartate

The liver is the center of nitrogen homeostasis through its synthesis of nitrogen-containing compounds (such as amino acids), its regulation of gluconeogenesis,

Table 1
Novel agents for treatment of hepatic encephalopathy with their mechanisms of action and clinical effects

Agent	Theorized Mechanism of Action	Clinical Effect
Acetyl carnitine	Supporting neuronal clearance of ammonia and free radicals	No clinical benefit observed despite reduced ammonia levels
Albumin	Reducing oxidation stress and inflammatory cascade	No improvement in overt HE; however, overall improvement in 3 mo mortality
AST-120	Preventing absorption of gut ammonia and toxins	No improvement in covert HE despite reduced ammonia levels
Flumazenil	Reducing GABAnergic response in neurons	Limited data suggest clinical benefit of short-term use
Fecal microbiota transplantation	Reducing peripheral inflammation through gut microbiome modification	Small trials demonstrate reduced hospitalizations for HE, but clinical applicability remains under investigation
Glycerol phenylbutyrate	Increasing urinary excretion of ammonia	Reduction in ammonia levels in phase II trials with reduced incidence of HE in follow-up studies
L-Ornithine L-aspartate	Increasing skeletal muscle use of ammonia	Reduction in HE grade in combination with lactulose
Polyethylene glycol	Increasing gut clearance of ammonia producing organisms	Improves mentation and reduces length of admission in patients hospitalized for HE compared with lactulose alone
Probiotics	Reducing peripheral inflammation through gut microbiome modification	Cochrane review found no benefit but overall poor data quality limited review

and the citric acid and urea cycles. Disruption of this homeostasis—as occurs in urea cycle disorders—results in accumulation of ammonia, which has toxic effects on the central nervous system at levels as low as 100 µmol/L and can lead to cerebral edema when levels exceed 1000 µmol/L.[5] Ammonia-scavenging agents have been used in urea cycle disorders to counteract these effects (**Fig. 1**).

The use of ammonia-scavenging agents to treat manifestations of liver disease originated with studies demonstrating the efficacy of phenylacetate in animal models of acute liver failure. Phenylacetate combined with L-ornithine (L-ornithine phenylacetate) works to clear serum ammonia via a 2-step process wherein ammonia is used by skeletal muscle to synthesize glutamine, with L-ornithine acting as a substrate in this pathway. Glutamine is subsequently excreted via urine, facilitated by phenylacetate as phenylacetateglutamine.[6] Several preliminary studies have demonstrated that ammonia-scavenging agents, including L-ornithine phenylacetate, reduce ammonia levels in cirrhotic patients.[6–8] A recent meta-analysis evaluating the clinical utility of L-ornithine in combination with L-aspartate (L-ornithine L-aspartate [LOLA]) concluded that LOLA was comparable with lactulose in both decreasing serum ammonia levels as well as improving clinical status, including mental state and

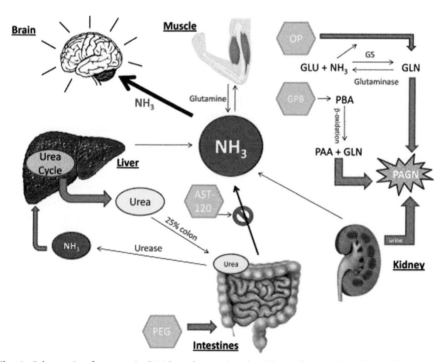

Fig. 1. Schematic of ammonia (NH_3) pathways involved in pathogenesis of HE with target sites of action for several novel agents. Polyethylene glycol (PEG) increases clearance of NH_3-synthesizing bacteria and AST-120 limits absorption of ammonia produced in the gut. Ornithine phenylacetate (OP) and glycerol phenylbutyrate (GPB) enhance clearance of NH_3 in urine by acting as substrates for glutamate synthetase (GS). Glutamate (GLU)-forming glutamine (GLN) and phenylacetate (PAA) work in conjunction to form phenylacetylglutamine (PAGN) before renal excretion. (*From* Rahimi RS, Rockey DC. Novel Ammonia-Lowering Agents for Hepatic Encephalopathy. *Clinics in liver disease.* 2015;19(3):539-549; with permission.)

electroencephalography activity, in patients with HE.[9] Similarly, a recent randomized controlled trial showed that, in combination with lactulose, LOLA at 30 g 3 times daily significantly decreased the grade of overt HE in cirrhotic patients not responsive to lactulose alone.[10] There are currently several NIH-funded clinical trials investigating the clinical utility of an oral formulation of L-ornithine in the prevention and management of HE.

Glycerolphenylbutarate

A prodrug of sodium phenylbutyrate, glycerolphenylbutarate (GPB), has been shown to be noninferior to sodium phenylacetate at lowering serum ammonia concentrations in patients with urea cycle disorders.[11] Similar to LOLA and other ammonia-scavenging agents, GPB facilitates clearance of ammonia through excretion of byproducts of its metabolism in the glutamate synthesis pathway. An open-label trial published in 2014 demonstrated that GPB effectively decreased circulating ammonia levels compared with placebo, and was both safe and well tolerated in cirrhotic patients with HE.[12]The authors further expanded on their preliminary studies in a phase II randomized controlled trial showing that treatment with GPB decreased incidence of HE among patients with decompensated cirrhosis more than placebo; these findings correlated with lower plasma ammonia levels in the GPB arm.[7]

Polyethylene Glycol

Before the introduction of lactulose as a therapeutic agent for HE, magnesium salts were the mainstay of therapy. The bowel cleansing action of these drugs was suspected to limit the amount of ammonia production by gut bacteria.[13,14] Following the adoption of lactulose, cathartic methods for managing HE were largely abandoned until a growing interest in the use of polyethylene glycol 3350-electrolyte solution (PEG) for patients hospitalized with overt encephalopathy. Following several smaller studies showing efficacy of PEG in HE,[15–18] the HELP (Hepatic Encephalopathy: Lactulose vs Polyethylene Glycol 3350-Electrolyte Solution) study randomized 186 patients to receive lactulose or PEG for the treatment of overt encephalopathy. This phase II study demonstrated greater improvement in mentation in the PEG group within 24 hours of treatment when compared with the lactulose arm. Patients in the PEG arm were noted to have reduced length of admissions and reduction in time required to resolve overt encephalopathy.[17]

Spherical Carbon Adsorbent

AST-120 is a carbon microsphere approved in Japan in 1991 for the management of uremic symptoms in nondialysis patients with chronic kidney disease. The microspheres are not absorbed and function by binding low molecular volume organic compounds within the gastrointestinal tract, and prevent gut absorption of toxins that cause encephalopathy.[16] In animal studies, AST-120 reduced ammonia levels, with more recent studies demonstrating an associated decrease in oxidative stress and neuroedema,[19] raising speculation that AST-120 may have a role in the management of HE. Phase II trials demonstrated findings similar to those in animal models; however, although AST-120 reduced serum ammonia levels, these findings did not translate to improved cognition in patients with covert HE. In a multicenter, double-blinded, randomized controlled trial, patients treated with AST-120 demonstrated a significant decline in serum ammonia levels, again without improved cognition.[20–22] Because of these results, further exploration into the role of AST-120 in HE has been limited.

GUT MICROBIOME MODULATORS
Fecal Microbiota Transplantation

Animal models of cirrhosis suggest that a disruption of the gut-hepatic-brain axis due to alterations in digestive tract flora and a resulting increase in the expression of proinflammatory cytokines and ammonia production contribute to the pathogenesis of HE.[23] Consistent with this hypothesis, cross-sectional and prospective studies have shown significant differences in the gut microbiome of patients with cirrhosis on and off lactulose and cirrhotic patients compared with matched, healthy controls.[23,24] It has been suggested that a compromised intestinal barrier contributes to systemic inflammation. This compromise facilitates translocation of pathogenic bacteria and subsequent endotoxemia resulting in an increased inflammatory milieu in the liver with increased systemic inflammation and neuroinflammation.[25–27]

Bajaj and colleagues[28] showed that cirrhotic patients had a colonic deficiency in bacteria belonging to autochthonous protective taxa, which have been shown to produce anti-inflammatory fatty acids and support the maintenance of the gut barrier.[29,30] These authors further demonstrated a correlation between cirrhotic decompensation and an increase in dysbiosis, as manifested by an overexpression of *Enterobacteriaceae* and *Bacteroidacea* species in the stool of subjects who developed HE. Similarly, unfavorable differences in the gut microbiome population are known to be associated with an abundance of proinflammatory serum markers, and have been shown to be especially pronounced in patients with HE, underscoring the importance of the inflammatory milieu associated with certain gut bacteria.[24,26]

As a result, several studies have investigated the protective role of the healthy, autochthonous gut flora on cognition in patients with cirrhosis. In recent years, fecal microbiota transplantation (FMT) has gained attention for its potentially beneficial effect on patients with gut dysbiosis. A widely accepted treatment of recurrent *Clostridium difficile* infection (rCDI), FMT involves the donation of fecal material from a healthy subject into a patient with presumed compromise of bacterial symbiosis in the gut, and has been associated with clinical resolution of rCDI at rates exceeding 80%.[31]

FMT was first purported as a viable treatment option for HE after a case report published in 2016 showed that serial FMT resulted in improved mentation in a patient admitted with HE, although the effect was transient and the treated patient had only had minimal HE, graded as a 1 to 2.[32] In a 2017 randomized clinical trial investigating the therapeutic effect of FMT in conjunction with lactulose and rifaximin among 10 patients versus 10 patients treated with lactulose and rifaximin alone; the FMT treatment arm had a statistically significant reduction in hospitalizations for recurrent HE and overall improved cognition.[33] This proof-of-concept study provided the framework for a subsequent randomized clinical trial with a similar sample size, without pretreatment antibiotics and using a capsule FMT option rather than an enema route; the authors demonstrated FMT to be safe and well tolerated with continued efficacy in long-term follow-up,[34] but the study was not powered to evaluate for efficacy of this modality in ameliorating HE. The clinical applicability of FMT for treating HE remains under investigation. Fortunately, there is extensive literature on the applicability of FMT in rCDI that can serve as guidance for future studies.

Probiotics

Similar to the therapeutic mechanism conferred by FMT, probiotics are proposed to exert a positive effect on HE by decreasing the burden of pathogenic intestinal bacteria promoting a healthy intestinal barrier and ameliorating the toxic effects of bacterial translocation in cirrhosis.[35–37] Most trials evaluating the applicability of probiotics in HE treatment involve VSL3 (also known as Visibiome), which has recently has been touted as an adjunct, dietary therapeutic for inflammatory bowel disease.[38] A combination of 8 strains of lactic acid-producing bacteria, including strains of *Lactobacillus*, *Bifidobacteria*, and *Streptococcus*, VSL3 has been shown to decrease bacterial translocation as well as serum tumor necrosis factor alpha (TNF-α) levels in experimental rat models of cirrhosis.[39] These findings were redemonstrated in adult patients with cirrhosis and minimal HE with mild cognitive impairment.[40] The authors noted a decrease in systemic markers of inflammation, including CRP and TNF-α in patients treated with VSL3 compared with placebo. In addition, measurement of surrogate serum markers of intestinal barrier compromise, including fatty acid-binding protein 6, were decreased in patients treated with VSL3, suggesting improved intestinal barrier integrity. These findings paralleled improvement in HE demonstrated by higher performance on cognitive testing.[40]

Despite ongoing, early phase studies alluding to the positive effect of probiotics, strong evidence supporting the use of probiotics to improve cognition in HE is lacking. A Cochrane review published in 2017 studied 21 trials, including more than 1400 participants evaluating the utility of probiotics in HE and concluded that probiotics likely did confer a benefit on HE by improving symptomology compared with no therapy or placebo; however, data were deemed low quality as most studies were fraught with bias.[41] Furthermore, despite their proposed effect on the gut-liver-brain axis, several studies have not found probiotics to alter the composition of the gut microbiome.[42–44] Of concern, probiotic research has raised concerns over potential adverse effects, including horizontal gene transfer of genetic material that confer antibiotic resistance.[45,46] Because the data for the use of probiotics in the treatment of HE are not robust, several ongoing studies aim to better understand the impact of this gut microbiome modulator on HE.

FLUMAZENIL

HE is characterized by an imbalance in excitatory and inhibitory neurotransmission in the central nervous system. Neurotransmission in patients with HE is predominately inhibitory, likely facilitated by hyperammonemia.[47–49] Gamma aminobutyric acid (GABA) is the main inhibitory neurotransmitter in the brain responsible for decreasing neuronal activity. Patients with HE are considered to have increased "GABAergic tone," rendering them attractive candidates for GABA/benzodiazepine receptor antagonists, such as flumazenil, which act by competitively binding to the benzodiazepine recognition site on this complex.[47]

Goh and colleagues[47] recently performed a recent meta-analysis of randomized clinical trials published from 1989 to 2009 to compare the effects of flumazenil versus placebo among patients with cirrhosis with varying degrees of HE severity, although most were diagnosed with overt HE. The efficacy of flumazenil versus placebo was determined by standard psychometric tests. Total intravenous flumazenil dosages ranged from 0.2 to 19.5 mg with treatment durations between 10 minutes and 72 hours.[47] The meta-analysis concluded that flumazenil had no impact on overall death rate, regardless of the cause, compared with placebo (mortality 7.4% vs 9.4% for treatment and placebo, respectively). There were insufficient data to assess adverse events; nor were there data on the effects of flumazenil on quality of life. Nevertheless, flumazenil treatment compared with placebo improved clinical symptoms of HE, albeit temporarily, when all trials were assessed. These findings were also demonstrated in a double-blind crossover clinical trial.[50]

At present, evidence for the beneficial short-term efficacy of flumazenil in treating patients with HE is limited. Although the meta-analysis suggested a short-term beneficial role in treating patients with HE, it found many limitations, including inappropriate study designs, lack of statistical rigor, and evidence of bias. In addition, a recent NIH trial of flumazenil in patients with HE was withdrawn due to insufficient recruitment. Because of these limitations, the use of flumazenil as a therapeutic option for HE remains unclear.

ACETYL CARNITINE

Unlike hepatocytes, astrocytes do not possess a urea cycle equivalent for clearance of ammonia.[51] Protection from the cellular insults that result from hyperammonemia in the brain, therefore, relies heavily on the glutamine synthase pathway, which uses glutamate and ammonia. However, studies have shown a dysregulation of the glutamine synthetase (GS) enzyme in hyperammonemic states, likely via inhibition of its activity by nitric oxide.[52] The downstream effect of GS disruption is accumulation of glutamine in the brain resulting in astrocyte swelling and death.[53,54]

Acetyl-L-carnitine (ACL) is an endogenous ester of L-carnitine that has been shown to lower ammonia levels in the blood and brain.[55–57] ACL is able to cross the blood-brain barrier where it donates its acetyl moiety for mitochondrial fatty acid oxidation and also acts as a substrate for the synthesis of membrane phospholipids and the production of cellular energy in astrocytes, thereby providing metabolic support for surrounding neurons.[58,59] Studies have also shown ACL to enhance the synthesis of acetylcholine esterase, giving rise to its candidacy as an adjunct therapy for slowing the progression of dementia.[60] ACL is purported to improve symptoms of HE by providing a neuronal cellular energy source for neurons, scavenging of free radicals and mitigating the excitotoxic effect of glutamate via its reduction of circulating ammonia levels through its role in urea synthesis.

In clinical trials evaluating ACL for mild to severe HE, Malaguarnera and colleagues[61,62] found that ACL, compared with placebo, improved symptoms of HE as assessed by neuropsychological testing and cognitive abilities, with parallel reductions in serum and brain ammonia levels. Neuropsychological testing and self-reporting of symptoms also revealed an improvement in mental and physical fatigue in patients with grade 3 HE.[63,64]

The clinical applicability of oral and intravenous formulations of this molecule as a therapy for HE was assessed in a 2019 Cochrane review of 5 studies comparing ACL with standard therapy. The review sought to assess the benefits and harms of ACL therapy in patients with HE and demonstrated a decrease in circulating ammonia plasma levels but no overall clinical benefit for ACL over placebo in ameliorating fatigue or quality of life. No data on the rate of side effects, hospital readmissions, or mortality were reported in any of the studies.[65] These findings contrasted with a non-Cochrane meta-analysis published by Jiang and colleagues[66] in 2013 that assessed the effect of oral ACL or L-carnitine on HE with the conclusion that ACL both decreased blood ammonia levels and improved cognitive function in HE compared with placebo, underscoring the need for further research involving ACL in HE.

ALBUMIN

The role of albumin as a possible therapeutic target for HE stems from its multiple potential functions in the human body. The most apparent is the effect of the protein on circulation and oncotic hemostasis. In addition, it also functions as a scavenger agent, reducing oxidative and nitrosative injury throughout the body, which have been impli-cated in the neuroedema associated with HE.[67,68] Earlier studies demonstrated the superiority of albumin compared with colloid in treatment of HE, supporting its role as a potential therapy.[69] Albumin does not seem to have a direct effect on the treat-ment of overt HE, however, does seem to improve overall mortality in patients with en-cephalopathy through its anti-inflammatory properties.[70–72] A recent randomized controlled study (N = 120) compared the use of combined lactulose plus albumin with lactulose alone in patients hospitalized for HE; the addition of albumin lowered serum levels of IL-6, IL-18, TNF-α, and endotoxin. Results also demonstrated reduced 3-month mortality despite a lack of reduction in HE.[71] Similar findings were also found in an earlier randomized double-blind study (N = 56 patients) that found improved survival at 90 days after a hospitalization for HE, again without any increased resolution of HE.[70]

ON THE HORIZON

As the understanding of the pathophysiology governing HE improves, further prom-ising therapeutic options continue to emerge. Studies on the catabolic effect of hyperammonemia on skeletal muscle highlight the mTOR signaling pathway as a po-tential therapeutic target,[73–75] especially given the potential role for sarcopenia in the pathogenesis of HE.[76–78] In fact, LOLA has been shown to mitigate the deleterious effect of hyperammonemia by reversing sarcopenia in animal models of cirrhosis.[79] Research regarding the GABAnergic pathway in HE is similarly prolific, with several animal studies advocating for neuroimmune modulators as potential therapeutics for HE.[80,81] Hernandez-Rabaza and colleagues[82] found overexpression of hippocampal GABA surface receptors in rat models of HE, and chronic treatment with the phos-phodiesterase type V inhibitor, sildenafil, normalized this overexpression via increased cGMP production. Malaguarnera and colleagues[80] demonstrated that bicuculline, a GABA receptor antagonist, had favorable effects on spatial learning in rat models of HE, likely via an inhibitory effect on neuroinflammation.[83] Similar findings were shown with other GABAnergic antagonists, including GR3027[81] and the anti-inflammatory sulforaphane.[84] In an animal model of cirrhosis, hydrogen sul-fide was also shown to ameliorate the neuroinflammatory cascade associated with hyperammonemia.[85]

Despite promising candidacy for several of these agents in treating HE, studies of their clinical applicability remain in the early phases, and in many instances with under-whelming results, underscoring the need for further, larger-scale investigations involving these novel therapies.

CONFLICTS OF INTEREST

S.C. Gordon receives grant/research support from AbbVie Pharmaceuticals, Conatus, CymaBay, Genfit, Gilead Sciences, Intercept Pharmaceuticals, and Merck. O. Sadiq and M. Alimirah have no conflicts of interest to declare.

REFERENCES

1. Vilstrup H, Amodio P, Bajaj J, et al. Hepatic encephalopathy in chronic liver dis-ease: 2014 practice guideline by the American association for the Study of Liver Diseases and the European Association for the Study of the Liver. Hepatology 2014;60(2):715–35.

2. Volk ML, Tocco RS, Bazick J, et al. Hospital readmissions among patients with decompensated cirrhosis. Am J Gastroenterol 2012;107(2):247–52.
3. Wong EL, Cheung AW, Leung MC, et al. Unplanned readmission rates, length of hospital stay, mortality, and medical costs of ten common medical conditions: a retrospective analysis of Hong Kong hospital data. BMC Health Serv Res 2011; 11:149.
4. Conn HO, Bircher J. Hepatic encephalopathy: management with lactulose and related carbohydrates. Michigan: Medi-Ed Pr; 1989.
5. De Las Heras J, Aldamiz-Echevarria L, Martinez-Chantar ML, et al. An update on the use of benzoate, phenylacetate and phenylbutyrate ammonia scavengers for interrogating and modifying liver nitrogen metabolism and its implications in urea cycle disorders and liver disease. Expert Opin Drug Metab Toxicol 2017;13(4): 439–48.
6. Ytrebo LM, Kristiansen RG, Maehre H, et al. L-Ornithine phenylacetate attenuates increased arterial and extracellular brain ammonia and prevents intracranial hypertension in pigs with acute liver failure. Hepatology 2009;50(1):165–74.
7. Rockey DC, Vierling JM, Mantry P, et al. Randomized, double-blind, controlled study of glycerol phenylbutyrate in hepatic encephalopathy. Hepatology 2014; 59(3):1073–83.
8. Misel ML, Gish RG, Patton H, et al. Sodium benzoate for treatment of hepatic encephalopathy. Gastroenterol Hepatol (N Y) 2013;9(4):219–27.
9. Butterworth RF, McPhail MJW. L-Ornithine L-aspartate (LOLA) for hepatic encephalopathy in cirrhosis: results of randomized controlled trials and meta-analyses. Drugs 2019;79(Suppl 1):31–7.
10. Sidhu SS, Sharma BC, Goyal O, et al. L-Ornithine L-aspartate in bouts of overt hepatic encephalopathy. Hepatology 2018;67(2):700–10.
11. Lichter-Konecki U, Diaz GA, Merritt JL 2nd, et al. Ammonia control in children with urea cycle disorders (UCDs); phase 2 comparison of sodium phenylbutyrate and glycerol phenylbutyrate. Mol Genet Metab 2011;103(4):323–9.
12. Ghabril M, Zupanets IA, Vierling J, et al. Glycerol phenylbutyrate in patients with cirrhosis and episodic hepatic encephalopathy: a pilot study of safety and effect on venous ammonia concentration. Clin Pharmacol Drug Dev 2013;2(3):278–84.
13. Manning RT, Delp M. Management of hepatocerebral intoxication. N Engl J Med 1958;258(2):55–62.
14. Dawson AM, Sherlock S, Summerskill WH. The treatment and prognosis of hepatic coma. Lancet 1956;271(6945):689–94.
15. Naderian M, Akbari H, Saeedi M, et al. Polyethylene glycol and lactulose versus lactulose alone in the treatment of hepatic encephalopathy in patients with cirrhosis: a non-inferiority randomized controlled trial. Middle East J Dig Dis 2017;9(1):12–9.
16. Rahimi RS, Rockey DC. Novel ammonia-lowering agents for hepatic encephalopathy. Clin Liver Dis 2015;19(3):539–49.
17. Rahimi RS, Singal AG, Cuthbert JA, et al. Lactulose vs polyethylene glycol 3350—electrolyte solution for treatment of overt hepatic encephalopathy: the HELP randomized clinical trial. JAMA Intern Med 2014;174(11):1727–33.
18. Shehata HH, Elfert AA, Abdin AA, et al. Randomized controlled trial of polyethylene glycol versus lactulose for the treatment of overt hepatic encephalopathy. Eur J Gastroenterol Hepatol 2018;30(12):1476–81.
19. Bosoi CR, Parent-Robitaille C, Anderson K, et al. AST-120 (spherical carbon adsorbent) lowers ammonia levels and attenuates brain edema in bile duct–ligated rats. Hepatology 2011;53(6):1995–2002.

20. Bajaj JS, Sheikh MY, Chojkier M, et al. Su1685 AST-120 (Spherical Carbon Adsorbent) in covert hepatic encephalopathy: results of the astute trial. Gastroenterology 2013;144(5):S-997.

21. Pockros P, Hassanein T, Vierling J, et al. 105 phase 2, multicenter, randomized study of ast-120 (spherical carbon adsorbent) vs. lactulose in the treatment of low-grade hepatic encephalopathy (HE). J Hepatol 2009;50:S43–4.

22. Zacharias HD, Zacharias AP, Gluud LL, et al. Pharmacotherapies that specifically target ammonia for the prevention and treatment of hepatic encephalopathy in adults with cirrhosis. Cochrane Database Syst Rev 2019;(6):CD012334.

23. Haussinger D, Schliess F. Pathogenetic mechanisms of hepatic encephalopathy. Gut 2008;57(8):1156–65.

24. Bajaj JS, Ridlon JM, Hylemon PB, et al. Linkage of gut microbiome with cognition in hepatic encephalopathy. Am J Physiol Gastrointest Liver Physiol 2012;302(1): G168–75.

25. Shawcross DL, Wright G, Olde Damink SW, et al. Role of ammonia and inflammation in minimal hepatic encephalopathy. Metab Brain Dis 2007;22(1):125–38.

26. Rai R, Saraswat VA, Dhiman RK. Gut microbiota: its role in hepatic encephalopathy. J Clin Exp Hepatol 2015;5(Suppl 1):S29–36.

27. Dhiman RK. Gut microbiota, inflammation and hepatic encephalopathy: a puzzle with a solution in sight. J Clin Exp Hepatol 2012;2(3):207–10.

28. Bajaj JS, Heuman DM, Hylemon PB, et al. Altered profile of human gut microbiome is associated with cirrhosis and its complications. J Hepatol 2014;60(5): 940–7.

29. Nava GM, Stappenbeck TS. Diversity of the autochthonous colonic microbiota. Gut Microbes 2011;2(2):99–104.

30. Dabard J, Bridonneau C, Phillipe C, et al. Ruminococcin A, a new lantibiotic produced by a *Ruminococcus gnavus* strain isolated from human feces. Appl Environ Microbiol 2001;67(9):4111–8.

31. Kelly CR, Kahn S, Kashyap P, et al. Update on fecal microbiota transplantation 2015: indications, methodologies, mechanisms, and outlook. Gastroenterology 2015;149(1):223–37.

32. Kao D, Roach B, Park H, et al. Fecal microbiota transplantation in the management of hepatic encephalopathy. Hepatology 2016;63(1):339–40.

33. Bajaj JS, Kassam Z, Fagan A, et al. Fecal microbiota transplant from a rational stool donor improves hepatic encephalopathy: a randomized clinical trial. Hepatology 2017;66(6):1727–38.

34. Bajaj JS, Fagan A, Gavis EA, et al. Long-term outcomes of fecal microbiota transplantation in patients with cirrhosis. Gastroenterology 2019;156(6):1921–3.e3.

35. Wiest R, Albillos A, Trauner M, et al. Targeting the gut-liver axis in liver disease. J Hepatol 2017;67(5):1084–103.

36. Soriano G, Guarner C. Probiotics in cirrhosis: do we expect too much? Liver Int 2013;33(10):1451–3.

37. Bajaj JS, Heuman DM, Hylemon PB, et al. Randomised clinical trial: *Lactobacillus* GG modulates gut microbiome, metabolome and endotoxemia in patients with cirrhosis. Aliment Pharmacol Ther 2014;39(10):1113–25.

38. Chapman TM, Plosker GL, Figgitt DP. Spotlight on VSL#3 probiotic mixture in chronic inflammatory bowel diseases. BioDrugs 2007;21(1):61–3.

39. Sanchez E, Nieto JC, Boullosa A, et al. VSL#3 probiotic treatment decreases bacterial translocation in rats with carbon tetrachloride-induced cirrhosis. Liver Int 2015;35(3):735–45.

40. Roman E, Nieto JC, Gely C, et al. Effect of a multistrain probiotic on cognitive function and risk of falls in patients with cirrhosis: a randomized trial. Hepatol Commun 2019;3(5):632–45.

41. Dalal R, McGee RG, Riordan SM, et al. Probiotics for people with hepatic encephalopathy. Cochrane Database Syst Rev 2017;(2):CD008716.

42. Kristensen NB, Bryrup T, Allin KH, et al. Alterations in fecal microbiota composition by probiotic supplementation in healthy adults: a systematic review of randomized controlled trials. Genome Med 2016;8(1):52.

43. Laursen MF, Laursen RP, Larnkjaer A, et al. Administration of two probiotic strains during early childhood does not affect the endogenous gut microbiota composition despite probiotic proliferation. BMC Microbiol 2017;17(1):175.

44. D'Mello C, Ronaghan N, Zaheer R, et al. Probiotics improve inflammation-associated sickness behavior by altering communication between the peripheral immune system and the brain. J Neurosci 2015;35(30):10821–30.

45. Wong A, Ngu DY, Dan LA, et al. Detection of antibiotic resistance in probiotics of dietary supplements. Nutr J 2015;14:95.

46. Zheng M, Zhang R, Tian X, et al. Assessing the risk of probiotic dietary supplements in the context of antibiotic resistance. Front Microbiol 2017;8:908.

47. Goh ET, Andersen ML, Morgan MY, et al. Flumazenil versus placebo or no intervention for people with cirrhosis and hepatic encephalopathy. Cochrane Database Syst Rev 2017;(8):CD002798.

48. Jones EA. Ammonia, the GABA neurotransmitter system, and hepatic encephalopathy. Metab Brain Dis 2002;17(4):275–81.

49. Hernandez-Rabaza V, Cabrera-Pastor A, Taoro-Gonzalez L, et al. Neuroinflammation increases GABAergic tone and impairs cognitive and motor function in hyperammonemia by increasing GAT-3 membrane expression. Reversal by sulforaphane by promoting M2 polarization of microglia. J Neuroinflammation 2016;13(1):83.

50. Barbaro G, Di Lorenzo G, Soldini M, et al. Flumazenil for hepatic encephalopathy grade III and IVa in patients with cirrhosis: an Italian multicenter double-blind, placebo-controlled, cross-over study. Hepatology 1998;28(2):374–8.

51. Rose C, Felipo V. Limited capacity for ammonia removal by brain in chronic liver failure: potential role of nitric oxide. Metab Brain Dis 2005;20(4):275–83.

52. Suarez I, Bodega G, Fernandez B. Glutamine synthetase in brain: effect of ammonia. Neurochem Int 2002;41(2–3):123–42.

53. Blei AT. Brain edema and portal-systemic encephalopathy. Liver Transpl 2000;6(4 Suppl 1):S14–20.

54. Braissant O, McLin VA, Cudalbu C. Ammonia toxicity to the brain. J Inherit Metab Dis 2013;36(4):595–612.

55. Therrien G, Rose C, Butterworth J, et al. Protective effect of L-carnitine in ammonia-precipitated encephalopathy in the portacaval shunted rat. Hepatology 1997;25(3):551–6.

56. Matsuoka M, Igisu H, Kohriyama K, et al. Suppression of neurotoxicity of ammonia by L-carnitine. Brain Res 1991;567(2):328–31.

57. Malaguarnera M, Pistone G, Elvira R, et al. Effects of L-carnitine in patients with hepatic encephalopathy. World J Gastroenterol 2005;11(45):7197–202.

58. Di Cesare Mannelli L, Ghelardini C, Toscano A, et al. The neuropathy-protective agent acetyl-L-carnitine activates protein kinase C-gamma and MAPKs in a rat model of neuropathic pain. Neuroscience 2010;165(4):1345–52.

59. Fiskum G, Rosenthal RE, Vereczki V, et al. Protection against ischemic brain injury by inhibition of mitochondrial oxidative stress. J Bioenerg Biomembr 2004;36(4): 347–52.

60. Yang Y, Choi H, Lee CN, et al. A multicenter, randomized, double-blind, placebo-controlled clinical trial for efficacy of acetyl-L-carnitine in patients with dementia associated with cerebrovascular disease. Dement Neurocogn Disord 2018; 17(1):1–10.

61. Malaguarnera M, Gargante MP, Cristaldi E, et al. Acetyl-L-carnitine treatment in minimal hepatic encephalopathy. Dig Dis Sci 2008;53(11):3018–25.

62. Malaguarnera M, Bella R, Vacante M, et al. Acetyl-L-carnitine reduces depression and improves quality of life in patients with minimal hepatic encephalopathy. Scand J Gastroenterol 2011;46(6):750–9.

63. Malaguarnera M, Vacante M, Giordano M, et al. Oral acetyl-L-carnitine therapy reduces fatigue in overt hepatic encephalopathy: a randomized, double-blind, placebo-controlled study. Am J Clin Nutr 2011;93(4):799–808.

64. Malaguarnera M, Vacante M, Motta M, et al. Acetyl-L-carnitine improves cognitive functions in severe hepatic encephalopathy: a randomized and controlled clinical trial. Metab Brain Dis 2011;26(4):281–9.

65. Marti-Carvajal AJ, Gluud C, Arevalo-Rodriguez I, et al. Acetyl-L-carnitine for patients with hepatic encephalopathy. Cochrane Database Syst Rev 2019;(1):CD011451.

66. Jiang Q, Jiang G, Shi KQ, et al. Oral acetyl-L-carnitine treatment in hepatic encephalopathy: view of evidence-based medicine. Ann Hepatol 2013;12(5):803–9.

67. Bernardi M, Ricci CS, Zaccherini G. Role of human albumin in the management of complications of liver cirrhosis. J Clin Exp Hepatol 2014;4(4):302–11.

68. Wright G, Jalan R. Ammonia and inflammation in the pathogenesis of hepatic encephalopathy: Pandora's box? Hepatology 2007;46(2):291–4.

69. Jalan R, Kapoor D. Reversal of diuretic-induced hepatic encephalopathy with infusion of albumin but not colloid. Clin Sci (Lond) 2004;106(5):467–74.

70. Simon-Talero M, Garcia-Martinez R, Torrens M, et al. Effects of intravenous albumin in patients with cirrhosis and episodic hepatic encephalopathy: a randomized double-blind study. J Hepatol 2013;59(6):1184–92.

71. Sharma BC, Singh J, Srivastava S, et al. Randomized controlled trial comparing lactulose plus albumin versus lactulose alone for treatment of hepatic encephalopathy. J Gastroenterol Hepatol 2017;32(6):1234–9.

72. Riggio O, Nardelli S, Pasquale C, et al. No effect of albumin infusion on the prevention of hepatic encephalopathy after transjugular intrahepatic portosystemic shunt. Metab Brain Dis 2016;31(6):1275–81.

73. Crossland H, Smith K, Atherton PJ, et al. The metabolic and molecular mechanisms of hyperammonaemia -and hyperethanolaemia-induced protein catabolism in skeletal muscle cells. J Cell Physiol 2018;233(12):9663–73.

74. Qiu J, Thapaliya S, Runkana A, et al. Hyperammonemia in cirrhosis induces transcriptional regulation of myostatin by an NF-kappaB-mediated mechanism. Proc Natl Acad Sci U S A 2013;110(45):18162–7.

75. Qiu J, Tsien C, Thapalaya S, et al. Hyperammonemia-mediated autophagy in skeletal muscle contributes to sarcopenia of cirrhosis. Am J Physiol Endocrinol Metab 2012;303(8):E983–93.

76. Dasarathy S. Consilience in sarcopenia of cirrhosis. J Cachexia Sarcopenia Muscle 2012;3(4):225–37.

77. Kalaitzakis E, Olsson R, Henfridsson P, et al. Malnutrition and diabetes mellitus are related to hepatic encephalopathy in patients with liver cirrhosis. Liver Int 2007;27(9):1194–201.

78. Kalaitzakis E, Bjornsson E. Hepatic encephalopathy in patients with liver cirrhosis: is there a role of malnutrition? World J Gastroenterol 2008;14(21):3438–9.

79. Kumar A, Davuluri G, Silva RNE, et al. Ammonia lowering reverses sarcopenia of cirrhosis by restoring skeletal muscle proteostasis. Hepatology 2017;65(6): 2045–58.

80. Malaguarnera M, Llansola M, Balzano T, et al. Bicuculline reduces neuroinflammation in hippocampus and improves spatial learning and anxiety in hyperammonemic rats. Role of glutamate receptors. Front Pharmacol 2019;10:132.

81. Johansson M, Agusti A, Llansola M, et al. GR3027 antagonizes GABAA receptor-potentiating neurosteroids and restores spatial learning and motor coordination in rats with chronic hyperammonemia and hepatic encephalopathy. Am J Physiol Gastrointest Liver Physiol 2015;309(5):G400–9.

82. Hernandez-Rabaza V, Agusti A, Cabrera-Pastor A, et al. Sildenafil reduces neuroinflammation and restores spatial learning in rats with hepatic encephalopathy: underlying mechanisms. J Neuroinflammation 2015;12:195.

83. Cauli O, Mansouri MT, Agusti A, et al. Hyperammonemia increases GABAergic tone in the cerebellum but decreases it in the rat cortex. Gastroenterology 2009;136(4):1359–67, e1-2.

84. Hernandez-Rabaza V, Cabrera-Pastor A, Taoro-Gonzalez L, et al. Hyperammonemia induces glial activation, neuroinflammation and alters neurotransmitter receptors in hippocampus, impairing spatial learning: reversal by sulforaphane. J Neuroinflammation 2016;13:41.

85. Kwon KW, Nam Y, Choi WS, et al. Hepatoprotective effect of sodium hydrosulfide on hepatic encephalopathy in rats. Korean J Physiol Pharmacol 2019;23(4): 263–70.

Moving?

Make sure your subscription moves with you!

To notify us of your new address, find your **Clinics Account Number** (located on your mailing label above your name), and contact customer service at:

Email: journalscustomerservice-usa@elsevier.com

800-654-2452 (subscribers in the U.S. & Canada)
314-447-8871 (subscribers outside of the U.S. & Canada)

Fax number: 314-447-8029

Elsevier Health Sciences Division
Subscription Customer Service
3251 Riverport Lane
Maryland Heights, MO 63043

*To ensure uninterrupted delivery of your subscription, please notify us at least 4 weeks in advance of move.